Essential Clinical Microbiology:
An Introductory Text

Essential Clinical Microbiology: An Introductory Text

E. M. Cooke, B.Sc., M.D., F.R.C.Path.,

Director of the Division of Hospital Infection,
Central Public Health Laboratory, Colindale, London, UK,
(formerly Professor of Clinical Microbiology,
University of Leeds, UK)

and

G. L. Gibson, M.D., F.R.C.Path.,

Director of the Public Health Laboratory, Leeds, and
Senior Clinical Lecturer, University of Leeds

A Wiley Medical Publication

JOHN WILEY & SONS
Chichester · New York · Brisbane · Toronto · Singapore

Copyright © 1983 by John Wiley & Sons Ltd.

Library of Congress Cataloging in Publication Data:

Cooke, Edith Mary.
  Essential clinical microbiology.
  (A Wiley medical publication)
  Includes index.
  1. Medical microbiology. I. Gibson, G. L. (George Lees) II. Title. III. Series. [DNLM: 1. Microbiological technics. 2. Microbiology. QW 4 C772c]
QR46.C78   1983   616′.01   82-11164
ISBN 0 471 90017 6

British Library Cataloguing in Publication Data:

Cooke, E. M.
  Essential clinical microbiology.
  1. Medical microbiology.
  I. Title. II. Gibson, G. L.
  616′.01   QR46
  ISBN 0 471 90017 6

Phototypeset by Dobbie Typesetting Service, Plymouth, Devon
Printed and bound in Great Britain at The Pitman Press, Bath

Preface

This book has arisen out of our experience of teaching medical students in Leeds during the past eight years. Microbiology is studied both in the pre-clinical period and then as part of the 'systems teaching' in the clinical course. We have felt the need for a text book which would give an adequate grounding in microbiology and have at the same time a clinical orientation. This book represents an attempt to meet this need.

Recognizing that many systems are affected by a wide variety of micro-organisms, we have included viruses, fungi, and protozoa as well as bacteria. The emphasis is on those diseases which are regularly seen in the United Kingdom, although exotic infections, rarer to us, are briefly included. We have attempted to meet the difficulties which students have expressed, and in order to promote familiarity with the large and daunting nomenclature of micro-organisms we have given the names of organisms in full on each occasion except when this would be too repetitious.

The principles of laboratory methods are stressed, but technical information is given only in sufficient detail to assist in the understanding of these principles. We hope that a reasonable knowledge of laboratory work may be gained so that useful clinical and laboratory liaison will be possible in later years.

We are indebted to our respective secretaries, Mrs E. Ellis and Mrs J. Brennan, who have been most patient and meticulous, and to Miss Renee Bailey for the great help she has given us by drawing the illustrations.

E. Mary Cooke
George L. Gibson

Contents

viii

Acknowledgements

Several of the figures in this book are adaptations of illustrations originally published elsewhere. The authors of this book wish to acknowledge that the following publications were used as reference sources for the creation of the figures listed below:

Figures 1.6, 1.7(a + b)–1.11: Chatterjee, K. D., 1962. *Parasitology, Protozoology and Helminthology in Relation to Clinical Medicine.* 4th Edition. Calcutta.

Figures 1.4, 1.5(a + c), 11.13b: Cruickshank, R., Duguid, J. P., and Swain, R. H. A., 1965. *Medical Microbiology.* 11th Edition. E. & S. Livingstone Ltd. Edinburgh and London.

Figure 1.12: Timbury, M C., 1975. *Notes on Medical Virology.* 5th Edition. Churchill Livingstone. Edinburgh, London and New York.

Figure 1.13: Duguid, J. P., Marmion, B. P., and Swain, R. H. A., 1978. *Medical Microbiology.* 13th Edition. Churchill Livingstone. Edinburgh, London and New York.

Figures 11.5 and 11.9: Gillies, R. R., and Dodds, T. C., 1976. *Bacteriology Illustrated.* 4th Edition. Churchill Livingstone. Edinburgh, London and New York.

Figure 16.9: Garrod, L. P., Lambert, H. P., and O'Grady, F. 1981. *Antibiotic and Chemotherapy.* 5th Edition. Churchill Livingstone. Edinburgh, London, Melbourne and New York.

CHAPTER I

Introduction

GENERAL CHARACTERISTICS OF MICRO-ORGANISMS

Micro-organisms are almost ubiquitous and show great variety in structure and activity. They ensure the fertility of the soil and the degradation of sewage. They are useful in the food, brewing, and pharmaceutical industries and more recently, as a consequence of genetic engineering, they have been used to synthesize complex therapeutic substances such as insulin.

The micro-organisms which cause disease and in which clinical microbiologists are interested form only a very small part of the total microbial population of the world. The fall into the Kingdom Protista, a large group of simple organisms. The protists can be further divided into:
   a) the higher protists which are eucaryocytic and which comprise the algae, protozoa, fungi, and slime moulds;
   b) the lower protists which are procaryocytic and which comprise the bacteria and the blue and green algae.

The procaryocytes are distinguished from the more complex eucaryocytes by:
   a) the possession of a simple nucleus with no nuclear membrane;
   b) the absence of internal membranes isolating separate enzyme systems;
   c) the possession of a rigid cell wall containing a specific mucopeptide.

Viruses are quite distinct from the organisms mentioned so far in that they reproduce only within living cells and contain DNA or RNA but not both. They must be considered as a separate group.

Bacteria

These are small procaryocytic structures which may have a variety of shapes. The cell consists of the genetic material and the cytoplasm, which is bounded by the cytoplasmic membrane and usually by a rigid cell wall. Other structures such as capsule, spore, flagella, and fimbriae may also be present (Fig. I,1).

Cytoplasm

This is a soft gel which contains the ribosomes. These are smaller than those of eucaryocytic organisms and are strung on strands of messenger RNA. The cytoplasm of some bacteria may also contain inclusion granules. These may consist of a variety of substances. They are usually energy stores and may be helpful in identification of the bacteria.

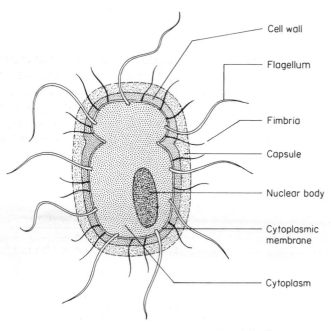

Figure I.1   The structure of the bacterial cell

Genetic material

The nucleus is a closed circle of double-stranded DNA. Bacteria replicate by binary fission, and because nuclear and cell division are not always synchronous, usually one but occasionally more nuclear bodies may be present. Additional genetic material may also be in the form of plasmids. These are small, usually circular, pieces of double-stranded DNA and they can replicate autonomously. They are smaller than the chromosome and are not essential to cell function. Plasmids are important in clinical microbiology because they may mediate for antibiotic resistance and also for properties associated with pathogenicity.

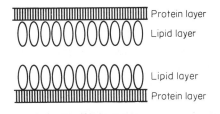

Figure I.2   The structure of the cell membrane

Cytoplasmic membrane

This limits the bacterial cytoplasm. Its structure is shown diagrammatically in Fig. I,2. Water diffuses passively through it, but inward transport of nutrients and outward transport of waste products is active. In Gram-positive organisms and less commonly in Gram-negative, invaginations of the cytoplasmic membrane called mesosomes occur. They may have a number of functions including the separation of the DNA between the daughter cells at cell division.

Cell wall

This is a rigid structure. It is complex, and because there is no counterpart in the eucaryocytic cells which make up human tissues it is the site of attack of some of the most effective and non-toxic antibiotics that are

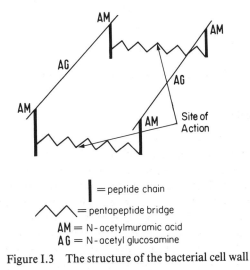

Figure I.3   The structure of the bacterial cell wall

available. For this reason an understanding of its structure is needed. The main structure is a mucopeptide consisting of N-acetyl glucosamine and N-acetylmuramic acid. The latter has a short peptide side chain. Chains are cross-linked by a peptide bridge which gives rigidity to the cell wall (Fig. 1,3). In Gram-positive organisms, although there are additional structures associated with the cell wall, these are relatively simple, but in Gram-negative organisms they may include lipopolysaccharide which is the endotoxin of the organism and may constitute a large proportion of the cell wall.

Spheroplasts are bacteria with an intact but weakened cell wall and protoplasts contain no cell wall. These rupture unless kept in solutions of high osmolarity.

L. forms and mycoplasmas are also bacteria with no cell wall.

Capsules

These surround some bacteria outside the cell wall and are usually composed of polysaccharide. Some capsulate organisms are surrounded by loose slime.

In some bacteria the capsule is small, can only be demonstrated serologically, and is known as a microcapsule. The capsule may protect against phagocytosis. Important capsulate organisms include pneumococci and klebsiellas.

Flagella

These are filamentous appendages and are the mechanism of locomotion in bacteria. Their number and distribution round the bacteria varies between species. Many medically important bacteria have flagella and are motile. These include pseudomonas, proteus, and salmonellas.

Fimbriae or pili

Fimbriae are fine hair-like structures surrounding some bacteria. They were first described in Gram-negative bacilli. They are shorter, finer, and more numerous than flagella and are organs of attachment. They may be of importance in pathogenicity.

Certain specialized fimbriae, 'sex fimbriae' or 'sex pili', take part in the transfer of DNA between bacteria in conjugation. They are longer than the common pili and are the site of attachment of specific phages, which are viruses which attack bacteria.

Spores

Sporulation is a complex activity resulting in the formation of structures which are able to remain dormant for long periods and to resist adverse conditions, particularly heat and absence of nutrients. Germination occurs when conditions are favourable and may be triggered by short periods of heat. Spores are of importance because they may allow organisms to survive for long periods and to be transferred for long distances, as for example with anthrax. Modern autoclaving, sterilizing, and canning procedures are all designed to destroy spores. In autoclaving, tetanus spores are particularly important and in canning, botulinus spores are the most important organisms which must be destroyed.

L forms and mycoplasmas

Both of these possess no cell wall and both may be cultured on cell-free media. L forms are often produced in the laboratory by exposure to penicillin. They are non-pathogenic but their persistence during penicillin administration may account for relapse following apparently successful therapy.

Mycoplasmas do not revert to the original bacterial form and they are pathogenic; the most important human pathogen is *Mycoplasma pneumoniae*.

Rickettsia, coxiella, and chlamydia

These are all bacteria but differ from most others by being obligate intracellular parasites. They must be distinguished from viruses from which they are quite separate. Typhus is an important rickettsial disease.

Fungi

These are non-photosynthetic eucaryocytic organisms with a rigid chitinous cell wall. They are divided into the moulds, which are filamentous mycelial fungi, and the unicellular yeasts. Yeast-like fungi grow partly as yeasts and partly as moulds and dimorphic fungi may exist as either according to the conditions. The systematic classification of fungi is based on their morphology, including the sporangium or spore-case borne on aerial hyphae and the macro- and micro-conidia which are also asexual spores. The structures of some of these of medical interest are shown in Fig. I,4. From the clinical point of view fungi are most

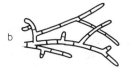

a

Macroconidia

b

Hyphae

Figure I.4   Some common fungal structures (Adapted from Cruikshank: *Medical Microbiology*, 12th Edition, by permission of Churchill Livingstone)

c

Hyphae with
microconidia

easily considered as candida spp., those causing systemic infections, and those dermatophytes which cause infections of the skin, hair and nails. They are discussed under these headings in Chapters 2, 9, and 11.

Viruses

These are quite different from the micro-organisms previously described, in that the genome consists of either DNA or RNA and this is reproduced within living host cells, where it directs the infected cell to produce the virion, the infective virus particle. This consists of the genome within a shell of protein, the capsid, which is composed of morphologically distinct units, the capsomeres. Some viruses also have an outer covering or envelope which is a lipo-protein and the whole virion has a defined symmetrical structure.

After a virion enters the host cell the capsid is removed and as a consequence of the presence of the viral nucleic acid, the host cell synthesises new viral nucleic acid, either DNA or RNA, and also the protein capsid. These are then assembled into new infectious particles which are released from the cell. Viruses are classified according to a number of properties particularly as to whether they contain RNA or

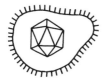

a Herpes Virus

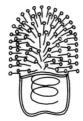

Figure I.5 Some common viral structures (a and c adapted from Cruikshank: *Medical Microbiology*, 12th Edition, by permission of Churchill Livingstone)

b Rhabdovirus

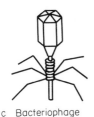

c Bacteriophage

DNA, their morphology, mode of transmission and the disease they cause (Fig. I,5).

Protozoa

These are unicellular non-photosynthetic eucaryocytic organisms. They are divided into four main groups and the mechanism of locomotion is important in the classification.

Mastigophora are flagellate, and trichomonads, giardia and trypanosomes are medically important flagellate protozoa (Fig. I,6). Amoeboid protozoa are the Rhizopoda and of these *Entamoeba histolytica*, a causative agent of dysentery, is the most important human pathogen of this group (Fig. I,7). Ciliated protozoa, the Ciliata, are of much less importance to man but the Sporozoa which have no organs of locomotion and have a complex life cycle include the plasmodium species, the causative agents of malaria (Fig. I,8).

8

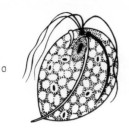

Trichomonas vaginalis

a

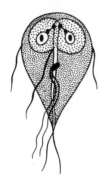

b

Figure I.6   Mastiogophora: Flagellate protozoa (adapted from Chatterjee: *Parasitology*, 4th Edition)

Giardia lamblia

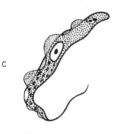

c

Trypanosome

Helminths

These are not Protists but belong to the Animal Kingdom. They are mentioned briefly here because they are important parasites of man and give rise to clinical syndromes which often resemble those caused by micro-organisms.

They are divided into the platyhelminths and the nemathelminths. (flat worms and round worms).

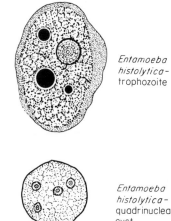

a   *Entamoeba histolytica-* trophozoite

b   *Entamoeba histolytica-* quadrinucleate cyst

Figure I.7   Rhizopoda: Amoeboid protozoa (adapted from Chatterjee: *Parasitology*, 4th Edition)

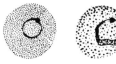

Ring forms of *Plasmodium vivax*

Female gametocyte of *Plasmodium vivax*

Male gametocyte of *Plasmodium falciparum*

Figure I.8   Sporozoa: Protozoa with a complex life cycle (adapted from Chatterjee: *Parasitology*, 4th Edition)

The platyhelminths include the cestodes and trematodes. Cestodes are tape-like and segmented; they are hermaphrodite with suckers and sometimes hooks on the head. Important cestodes or tape worms include the beef tape worm, *Taenia saginata*, the pork tape worm, *Taenia solium*, and the causative agent of hydatid disease, *Taenia echinococcus* (*Echinococcus granulosus*, Fig. I,9).

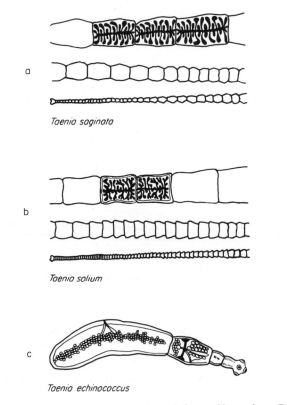

Figure I.9   Cestodes: Tape worms (adapted from Chatterjee: *Parasitology*, 4th Edition)

The trematodes are leaf-like, unsegmented and usually hermaphrodite. The head has suckers and there is an incomplete alimentary tract. The schistosoma are trematodes and are blood flukes which are important pathogens of man in many parts of the world (Fig. I,10). Liver and intestinal flukes are also trematodes.

Nematodes are elongated, cylindrical, and unsegmented. There are distinct sexes. There are no hooks or suckers and the alimentary canal

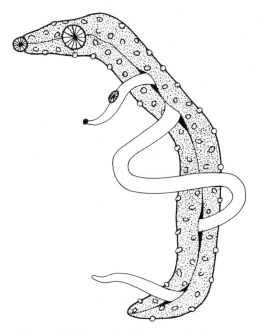

Mature adult worms of *Schistosoma haemotobium* as they exist in vesical venous plexus

Figure I.10   Trematodes: Flukes (adapted from Chatterjee: *Parasitology*, 4th Edition)

is complete. Important nematodes include the hookworms, *Ankylostoma duodenale* and *Necator americanus*. These are called hookworms because the anterior end of the worm is bent or hooked. The threadworm, *Enterobius vermicularis*, the filariae and many other human pathogens are nematodes (Fig. I,11).

COMMENSALS AND PATHOGENS

Those bacteria normally present on the body and not normally causing disease are referred to as commensals. Pathogens are those organisms which regularly cause disease in normal individuals.

Both these types of organisms are parasites, that is, they obtain nourishment from a living host. The term parasite is also used in relation to larger organisms, protozoa and helminths which are only briefly discussed in this book.

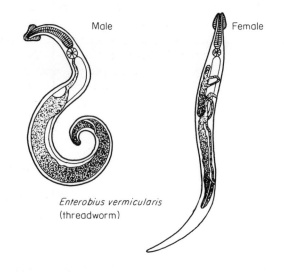

Male

Female

Enterobius vermicularis
(threadworm)

Figure I.11   Nematodes: Round worms. (adapted from Chatterjee: *Parasitology*,
4th Edition)

Recently much interest has centred on a group of organisms described as opportunistic pathogens or opportunists. These are organisms which may be commensal in one site but pathogenic in another and which will cause disease when the defences of the host are reduced. Bacteria such as *E. coli* and klebsiellas normally present in the gut, regularly act as opportunists. The factors contributing to this include the complexity of modern surgical procedures, the administration of cytotoxic drugs and the presence of severe underlying disease. Opportunistic infections are now of major importance.

NORMAL FLORA

The ubiquity of micro-organisms is reflected in the colonization of all surfaces of the body and of the gut.

The skin flora consists of coagulase negative staphylococci and propionobacteria (anaerobic diphtheroids). In addition, transient organisms will remain for short periods of time.

The mouth flora is extremely complex; amongst many other organisms present are viridans streptococci, corynebacteria, bacteroides spp., and borrelia. In health the stomach and small bowel have a limited microbial flora but the distal few inches of the small bowel and the large bowel are heavily colonized. Numerically by far the greatest population is anaerobic. Bacteroides spp., anaerobic cocci, and lactobacilli are present and in smaller numbers clostridia, particularly *Clostridium perfringens*. The aerobic population includes a variety of Gram-negative bacilli. *Escherichia coli* is almost always present and in some individuals proteus, pseudomonas or klebsiellas will be found. Streptococci (*Streptococcus faecalis*, enterococci) are regularly present.

The normal flora of the vagina is also complex. The lactobacilli present act on glycogen to produce lactic acid and maintain a low pH during the reproductive period of life. As well as lactobacilli, group B streptococci, anaerobic cocci, and a variety of other organisms may be present.

The normal flora of the body is important in preventing the establishment of pathogens. It may be markedly changed in disease and as a consequence of antibiotic usage.

GROWTH AND NUTRITION OF MICRO-ORGANISMS

Generally the aim in the laboratory is to produce environmental conditions which will enable as many as possible of the human pathogens in which we are interested to grow.

Bacteria

Most of the bacteria that are of medical interest are cultured at body temperature. There are some exceptions: for example, some skin pathogens grow at lower temperatures and a few bacteria, such as campylobacter spp., which grow at 43°C, require a higher temperature.

The atmosphere in which incubation is carried out is also important. Many bacteria are aerobic, that is they grow in the presence of oxygen. They may also be facultative anaerobes able to grow in the absence of air. Strict anaerobes will only grow in the absence of oxygen. Important human pathogens such as *Clostridium tetani*, the causative agent of tetanus, and bacteroides spp. which cause post-operative infections are strict anaerobes. There has been, during the last few years, a great increase in awareness of the importance of anaerobes in hospital infections.

Some bacteria require additional carbon dioxide for growth. Gonococci are a good example of this.

Bacteria may be cultured in liquid or solid media. Nutrient is usually provided by a protein hydrolysate and additional growth factors from other sources such as blood, serum or egg, may be added. The aim in diagnostic work is to provide the conditions which will allow isolation of the widest possible variety of important pathogenic organisms. The media used are those which will allow this.

Selective media

It may be desirable in some circumstances to promote the growth of one particular organism from amongst many that are present in the specimen. This most often occurs when examining faeces for intestinal pathogens, although it does occur in other situations also. Selective media are solid media that contain substances which inhibit some organisms but allow the pathogen in which we are interested to grow. An example of a selective medium is deoxycholate agar which is used for the isolation of dysentery bacilli. On it *Shigella* spp. grow quite well but *E. coli* and other intestinal bacteria are inhibited.

Enrichment media

Enrichment media are liquid media that allow some organisms to multiply faster than others. This may be achieved by adding substances that inhibit unwanted organisms or those that favour the multiplication of the pathogen. Selenite broth is an enrichment medium in which salmonellas multiply much faster than coliforms. Salmonellas present in small numbers can, therefore, be isolated from faeces containing many other organisms.

Indicator media

Some media undergo visible changes due to the activity of certain bacteria. These are indicator media. MacConkey agar contains lactose and an indicator. Organisms which ferment lactose produce acid which turns the indicator red. This is useful in distinguishing lactose fermenting coliforms, which are generally non-pathogenic in the gut, from salmonellas and shigellas which are non-lactose fermenters and are pathogenic.

Some bacteria, particularly the rickettsiae and chlamydiae, can only be cultured on living cells. Techniques similar to those for viruses are used.

A few bacteria cannot be cultured at all outside the living animal. Human pathogens of this sort include *Mycobacterium leprae* and *Treponema pallidum*, the causative agents of leprosy and syphilis.

Fungi

These are cultured on solid media in a similar way to bacteria, although the media used are generally those which will allow fungi to grow but which will suppress the growth of bacteria. Many fungi, particularly those causing skin diseases, grow best at 26–28°C.

Viruses

These require living cells for growth. They may be cultured in the living animal, the fertile egg or in cell culture. Living animals are not extensively used but are occasionally necessary, as in the use of suckling mice for Coxsackie virus.

Fertile hens' eggs may be inoculated on to the chorio-allantoic membrane or into the amniotic allantoic or yolk sacs (Fig. I,12). They have been particularly used for the isolation of pox-viruses and herpes-viruses.

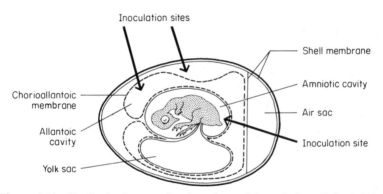

Figure I.12 Fertile hen's egg showing sites of inoculation (Adapted from Timbury: *Notes on Medical Virology*, 7th Edition, by permission of Churchill Livingstone)

Cell cultures may be produced from almost any normal tissues by trypsinization. The cells will grow if surrounded by nutrient media. They are in the form of monolayer and will continue to divide for a number of generations, although they eventually die. Some cell lines, particularly those such as HeLa cells derived from carcinomatous tissue, will multiply indefinitely.

Cell cultures are extensively used in diagnostic virology. The growth of the virus may be demonstrated by the visible effect it produces on the cells (the cytopathic effect), but sometimes the virus may grow without producing any obvious effect and other techniques to demonstrate its presence are required.

Protozoa

The diagnosis of protozoal infections is generally made by demonstrating the presence of the protozoa in suitable clinical material by direct microscopy. Serological investigations may also be used, particularly to demonstrate past infection. However, many protozoa may be cultured in the laboratory using simple liquid or solid media often similar to those used for bacterial culture. For example, trypanosomes can be cultured on blood agar slopes and trichomonads under anaerobic conditions in an isotonic medium containing, amongst other things, liver digest, calf serum and antibiotics.

SOURCES AND METHODS OF SPREAD OF INFECTIONS

Sources

The sources of infection may be exogenous or endogenous.

Exogenous infections of man may be contracted from animals or the environment, but the most common source is another person carrying the pathogen. This person may be suffering from the disease or he may be a symptomless carrier. Carriers are important in the spread of some diseases such as diphtheria and typhoid. They may never show symptoms of the disease or the symptoms may be so mild as to go unrecognized. Convalescent carriers are seen in some conditions, particularly salmonella infections.

A number of diseases are predominantly infections of animals. Spread to man is occasional and man-to-man spread may be rare or may never occur. Examples are brucellosis and salmonella food poisoning. In some situations, once spread to the human population has occurred, man-to-man spread does take place, as for example in pneumonic plague and yellow fever.

Other infections are spread to man directly from the environment. For example, *Clostridium tetani* is found in soil and may infect man if soil contaminates a wound. The source of the organism in the soil is originally the gut of an herbivorous animal. *Legionella pneumophila* is found in contaminated water and may spread to man via showers or humidification systems.

Endogenous infections of man arise from organisms carried by the patient himself. The urinary tract is infected by the patient's own bowel organisms. Many opportunistic infections arise in this way.

Methods of Spread

Infection may spread to man via a variety of routes and an understanding of the methods of spread of micro-organisms is an essential step in the control of the diseases that they cause.

Respiratory infections

These are spread by direct contact, by contaminated articles, by the inhalation of contaminated dust and sometimes by very small particles, droplet nuclei, which are expelled from the mouth of an infected patient (Fig. I,13).

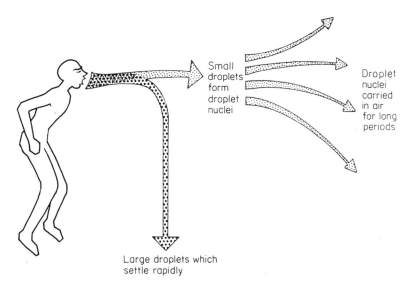

Figure I.13   Large and small droplets and droplet nuclei which spread respiratory infection (Adapted from Mackie and McCartney: *Medical Microbiology*, 13th Edition, by permission of Churchill Livingstone)

Infections of the skin

These occur particularly if the integrity of the skin has been breached. They may occur by direct contact with hands or clothing, or particularly in the case of burns and hospital wound infection, by exposure to airborne particles or pathogen-containing droplet spray from the mouths of attendants.

Venereal infections

These are spread by sexual contact and they are caused by organisms such as *Trepomena pallidum* and *Neisseria gonorrhoeae* which will not survive outside the body except for very short periods. Under very poor hygienic conditions these infections may be spread non-venereally.

Alimentary tract infections

These may be spread by the method usually rather unpleasantly described as the faecal–oral route. Infective hepatitis is an important disease which may be spread in this way. The route may be indirect and involve faecal contamination of water supplies such as occurs in outbreaks of cholera and typhoid, or contamination of food from the hands of a carrier, by flies, or in other ways, may occur.

Infection by direct inoculation

In some diseases spread takes place by direct inoculation through the patient's skin. This may accidentally occur in hospitals via syringe-needles, and serum hepatitis may occasionally be spread in this way. Blood-sucking arthropods spread diseases such as malaria, plague and typhus.

MECHANISMS OF DISEASE PRODUCTION

Once micro-organisms have reached the host, they must, if they are to produce disease, be able to breach the skin or mucous membrane. Usually they fail to do so but if, however, they succeed, they must next be able to establish themselves and cause disease. The ability of an organism to do all these things and also the severity of the disease produced are often referred to under the general term "virulence". The whole subject of bacterial virulence is complex and poorly understood, but undoubtedly the production by bacteria of toxins and enzymes is important.

Some bacterial exotoxins are elaborated by the bacteria and then act remotely from the site of infection. Bacteria which produce potent exotoxins include diphtheria and tetanus bacilli. Endotoxins are also important but are different in a number of ways. They are typically found in Gram-negative bacilli where they form part of the bacterial cell wall and are only released when the bacteria are disrupted. Endotoxins are potent pyrogens. Endotoxic shock occurs in man when there is a sudden release of endotoxin into the circulation, as may occur in septicaemia. There is fever, a marked fall in blood pressure and the condition may be fatal.

Bacteria may also produce enzymes which may be important in the pathogenesis of disease. Coagulase is produced by *Staphylococcus aureus* and helps the organism to establish itself by forming a fibrin barrier round it and preventing phagocytosis. Hyaluronidase dissolves the substance that binds the cells together and allows spread of the organism. Many other enzymes have been described which may be of importance in bacterial pathogenecity.

As well as the production of toxins and enzymes, the ability of some organisms to cause severe infections is clearly related to the ability of the organisms to spread within the body. *Streptococcus pyogenes* for example resists phagocytosis and causes a spreading infection, and some organisms, such as tubercle bacilli, are readily phagocytosed but are not destroyed within the phagocyte. Capsules are important in enabling organisms to resist phagocytosis.

In spite of those various mechanisms of pathogenicity, host defences against infection are generally so good that, certainly in developed countries, many people suffer little more than inconvenience from infection throughout most of their lives. These host defences will now be described.

HOST DEFENCES AGAINST INFECTION

General aspects of immunity to infection

The ability of a micro-organism to produce disease depends in part on its 'virulence' and in part on the ability of the host to resist infection by that particular pathogen.

These are marked species differences in microbial pathogenicity and although animals may be a source of some human infections many animal infections never spread to man at all. Also within the human species there are variations between races in their susceptibility to infection quite apart from those related to living conditions. These genetic differences are presumably related to past experience or lack of experience of the disease. The high susceptibility of American Indians to tuberculosis is an example. Within races there are individual differences in susceptibility. This is exemplified by the high incidence of similar infections in homozygous but not heterozygous twins.

Age may affect immunity to disease and some infections are more common and more severe at the extremes of life. Sex differences in susceptibility to infection are not marked. There is, however, good evidence that poor nutrition contributes to susceptibility to infectious disease.

Individual immunity to infection

Host defences against infection are divided into those which are non-specific and unrelated to prior experience of the infecting agent and those specific responses based on the development of acquired immunity.

Non-specific or 'innate' immunity

The mechanical barriers to infection are the skin and mucous membranes, both of which, as well as providing an intact barrier, have a variety of additional mechanisms which prevent ingress of bacteria. In the case of skin the lactic acid and fatty acids produce a low pH which results in the death after a short time of most organisms when put on the skin. Mucus has a protective effect and mechanical devices such as cilia in the respiratory tract and the washing action of urine in the urinary tract are also important. The large number of commensal organisms on the skin and in the bowel act by competing for nutrients and by producing inhibitory substances such as bacteriocins.

Lysozyme is present in many secretions, particularly tears, and will lyse many Gram-positive bacteria. Viral infections result in the production of interferon, a non-specific anti-viral agent which prevents infection with a second unrelated virus and aids in recovery from viral infections.

Once micro-organisms gain access to the body a complex series of reactions develop which often result in phagocytosis and digestion of the micro-organism by phagocytes. The 'alternative complement pathway' is activated by microbial surface carbohydrates. C_3 convertase is produced, C_3b binds to the surface of the organism, and C_3a attracts the polymorphs. These then become attached to the micro-organism by virtue of their C_3b receptors and ingestion follows.

Specific or acquired immunity

This may be passive or active.

Passive immunity

Passive immunity may be naturally acquired from the mother or may be artificially acquired. Preformed maternal antibody passes to the infant and provides protection for the first few months of life.

The administration of anti-tetanus serum containing antibodies to help prevent tetanus, or of γ-globulin to protect against infective hepatitis are examples of passive artificial immunity, used in the prophylaxis of infection. Passive immunity is short-lived as the γ-globulin preformed by another individual or even another species is destroyed fairly quickly in the recipient's body.

Active immunity

This is produced by exposure to infection or by immunization with a live or killed vaccine (Chapter XVIII).

Antibodies are produced by B lymphocytes; the antigen reacts with antibody already on the lymphocyte surface and this 'selected' lymphocyte is stimulated so that a large population of lymphocytes producing antibody and a population of memory cells are formed. Because of this the active production of antibody to an infecting organism is very much greater and more rapid on the second exposure of the host to the antigen. Demonstration of a rise in antibody level is often used in the diagnosis of infections, particularly those in which isolation of the infecting organism is difficult. There are also differences in the type of antibody produced at different stages of infection. IgM antibody is present during the acute phase of the disease and IgG antibody appears later. This is important as it enables one to distinguish whether an infection is recent or not. Other immunoglobulins are also important. IgA is found in secretions such as tears and saliva, in the gastro-intestinal and respiratory tracts. It forms part of the protection of the exposed surfaces of the body against microbial attack.

The role of IgE is less clear but it is known that the serum level rises in helminthic infections and it may provide protection against these parasites.

Antibody mediated immunity may function by opsonization, that is by coating of the infecting organism. Such coated bacteria adhere to phagocytes which will then engulf and digest them. In addition, the classical complement pathway is activated so that chemotaxis of the polymorphs to the coated bacteria occurs.

Antibodies may also function by neutralization of specific toxins produced by bacteria, and antibodies in the presence of complement may cause lysis of Gram-negative bacilli.

T-cell mediated, acquired cellular immunity is important in a number of conditions, particularly tuberculosis and brucellosis. Enhancement of macrophage activity occurs if there has been previous exposure of the host to the organism. The cells may become more actively phagocytic and intracellular growth of the organism is inhibited. This type of response, which is a delayed hypersensitivity reaction, is demonstrated by the tuberculin test when positive (Chapter XVIII).

In viral infections, antibody mediated immunity is important in those infections in which the virus passes through the blood stream and IgA antibody is particularly important in diseases of the respiratory tract. Cell mediated immunity is probably less important in viral diseases although it does play a part as shown by the ability of children with congenital hypogammaglobulinaemia to recover from infection.

Some parasitic infections are relatively insusceptible to the immune response, partly due to antigenic variation and partly because of the complexity of the life cycle of the parasite with different antigenic determinants associated with each phase. For these reasons immunization against parasitic diseases is little used, although there are hopes that a vaccine against malaria may become available before too long.

There are a number of clinical conditions in which immunoglobulin synthesis is impaired or cell mediated responses are reduced and patients suffering from these are highly susceptible to certain infections.

BACTERIAL GENETICS

Bacterial DNA is in the form of a closed coiled circle. At replication, the DNA strands in the helix separate and complementary strands are formed so that the offspring of cell division are identical. Possibilities of change are provided by mutation, with the mutants surviving if the mutation confers a selective advantage on the bacteria. Change may also be introduced by the transfer of genetic material between bacteria and for this three mechanisms exist: transformation, transduction, and conjugation.

Transformation

This involves the uptake of free DNA directly from the environment of the bacteria (Fig. I,14). The DNA must have been derived from a closely related species. The classical experiments on transformation involved the transfer of DNA mediating for capsule production between strains of pneumococci, but transfer also occurs between *Haemophilus influenzae* strains and *Bacillus* species.

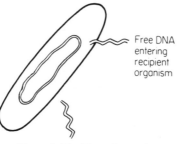

Figure I.14   Transformation

Transduction

Generalized and restricted transduction and lysogenic conversion must be considered.

Generalized transduction

The transfer of bacterial genes by phages results in generalized transduction. The bacterial genes replace the normal phage genome in the phage head and the transferred genes may be incorporated into the host cell chromosomes by recombination (Fig. I,15). Usually chromosomal genes are transferred but extrachromosomal DNA (plasmids) may also be transduced. Penicillinase production in staphylococci may be transferred by this type of transduction.

Restricted transduction

This is also phage-mediated but involves the transfer of a much smaller amount of bacterial DNA. Phages that infect bacteria may be virulent and result in lysis of the host cell. However, many phages are temperate and become latent in the cell. In this situation multiplication of the phage is repressed and the phage is incorporated into the bacterial

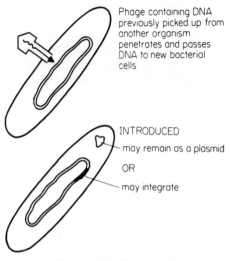

Phage containing DNA previously picked up from another organism penetrates and passes DNA to new bacterial cells

INTRODUCED

may remain as a plasmid

OR

may integrate

Figure I.15   Transduction

chromosome. If the repression is lifted, the phage is excised. This excision may be inaccurate and a small proportion of the bacterial DNA may be excised as well. When the phage genome is integrated into a second cell, the small piece of bacterial DNA is also integrated and reproduced in the progeny of other cells. This is restricted transduction.

Lysogenic conversion

The presence of the lysogenic prophage DNA in bacteria may, however, be important for reasons other than those mentioned so far. Occasionally prophage genes are expressed and confer new properties on the cell. This is lysogenic conversion and an interesting example is the production of toxin by *Corynebacterium diphtheriae* which only occurs when the diphtheria bacillus is lysogenized by phage.

Conjugation

Many bacteria contain plasmids. These are small pieces of extrachromo-somal DNA that replicate autonomously. They usually code for properties that are not essential but are useful under certain circumstances. The most important ones from a medical point of view code for antibiotic resistance and for some virulence factors such as enterotoxin production. During conjugation the donor transfers genetic material directly to

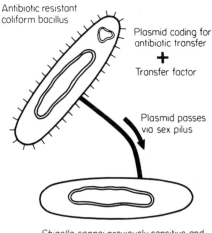

Antibiotic resistant
coliform bacillus

Plasmid coding for
antibiotic transfer

+

Transfer factor

Plasmid passes
via sex pilus

Shigella sonnei previously sensitive and
now antibiotic resistant

Figure I.16   Conjugation

the recipient. To be able to do this the donor organism must contain a transmissible plasmid, that is one that is autonomously transferrable due to the presence of a transfer factor. These transfer factors code for the production of sex fimbriae or pili. These are longer and finer than common pili. The pilus may hold the two cells together but the actual mechanism of DNA transfer is not clear (Fig. I,16).

Some transfer factors, notably the F factor in *E. coli*, may become integrated into the bacterial chromosome. Such cells are known as Hfr cells as they are able to transfer chromosomal genes into F^- cells at a high frequency. Not only may the F factor be transferred, but also adjacent portions of the chromosome to which it is attached.

There are many types of bacterial plasmids. As stated, they may be transmissible as they contain transfer factors. They may also code for antibiotic resistance. As transfer occurs between different species of bacteria and as plasmids may code for multiple antibiotic resistance, the implications for development and spread of antibiotic resistant bacteria are obvious. One surprising consequence of this mechanism of antibiotic resistance is that use of one antibiotic may select for strains resistant not only to that antibiotic but resistant to others also and that this resistance may be distributed in several bacterial species. A good example of the transfer of multiple antibiotic resistance is between *E. coli* and *Shigella* species.

CHAPTER II

The Major Groups
of Human Pathogens

In this chapter is summarized information about the micro-organisms commonly associated with disease in man. They are considered in the following order: bacteria, viruses, fungi, and protozoa.

BACTERIA

These include Gram-positive and Gram-negative cocci and bacilli, vibrios, spirochaetes, chlamydiae and rickettsiae.

Gram-positive cocci

These are staphylococci and micrococci in which the cocci are in clusters, and the streptococci in which they are arranged in chains (Fig. II,1).

Staphylococci and micrococci

Staphylococcus aureus (Staphylococcus pyogenes)

This is the major human pathogen in this group. The name 'aureus' is given because many of the strains produce golden colonies on solid media in the laboratory. It is distinguished from other staphylococci and micrococci by the production of a number of enzymes and toxins, the most important of which is coagulase (Fig. II,2). Most coagulase positive organisms are also DNase and phosphatase positive. It is carried in the anterior nares of about 50% of normal people and on the skin of about 10% and is an important cause of infection in man, particularly in hospitals. Diseases caused include boils, whitlows, wound infection, osteomyelitis and rarely pneumonia and enterocolitis. Initially sensitive to many antibiotics, now many strains are resistant to penicillin and tetracycline, but usually sensitive to cloxacillin, gentamicin, and fucidin. Staphylococci are typed by their sensitivity to phages. These are viruses

GRAM STAIN

The Gram stain and the morphology of the organisms form the basis of a simple classification of common bacteria. The organisms are stained by methyl violet fixed with iodine. When ethyl alcohol is applied some bacteria retain the stain, appear dark blue, and are described as Gram positive. Some lose their methyl violet stain, become colourless and when counterstained with dilute carbol fuchsin appear pink. These are described as Gram negative.

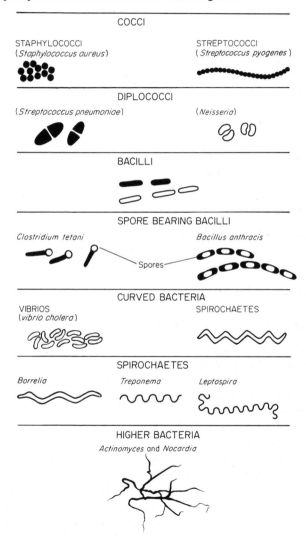

Figure II.1   Classification of bacteria by Gram-staining and morphology

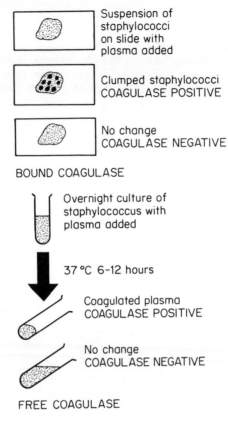

Suspension of
staphylococci
on slide with
plasma added

Clumped staphylococci
COAGULASE POSITIVE

No change
COAGULASE NEGATIVE

BOUND COAGULASE

Overnight culture of
staphylococcus with
plasma added

37 °C 6-12 hours

Coagulated plasma
COAGULASE POSITIVE

No change
COAGULASE NEGATIVE

FREE COAGULASE

Figure II.2   Coagulase test

which are parasitic upon them and which cause bacterial lysis (Fig. II,3). This is valuable in studying hospital outbreaks of infection (Chapter XIV).

Staphylococcus albus (Staphylococcus epidermidis)

This is called 'albus' because many strains produce white colonies. It is coagulase negative. It is widely distributed on normal skin, and non-pathogenic except as a cause of infection in immunologically compromised individuals and of endocarditis following open heart surgery.

Micrococci

These are similar to the coagulase negative staphylococci. Some strains of micrococci cause urinary tract infection.

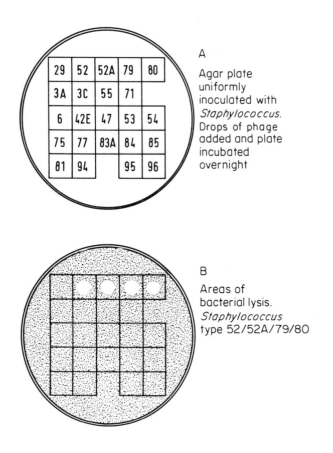

A

Agar plate
uniformly
inoculated with
Staphylococcus.
Drops of phage
added and plate
incubated
overnight

B

Areas of
bacterial lysis.
Staphylococcus
type 52/52A/79/80

Figure II.3   Phage typing

Streptococci

These are subdivided according to their haemolytic reactions on blood agar plates and their antigenic structure.

Streptococci may be:

β haemolytic — producing complete haemolysis;

α haemolytic — producing partial greenish haemolysis;

γ haemolytic — producing no haemolysis.

The antigens studied are the polysaccharide components of the cell wall (Lancefield grouping) and the protein surface structures (Griffith typing).

The clinically important streptococci are *Streptococcus pyogenes, viridans streptococci, Streptococcus faecalis, Streptococcus pneumoniae,* and anaerobic streptococci.

Streptococcus pyogenes

This is a β haemolytic streptococcus of Lancefield Group A. It is an important human pathogen and is carried in the throat of 5% and the nose of 1% of normal individuals. The diseases associated with *Streptococcus pyogenes* include those directly due to the infecting organism and the delayed sequelae of infection.

The acute infections include tonsillitis which may spread locally causing acute otitis media and mastoiditis. Scarlet fever occurs when tonsillitis is caused by a strain of the organism which produces an erythrogenic toxin giving rise to a generalized rash. Erysipelas is a true skin infection; burns and wounds may also be infected while rarely puerperal sepsis may be due to streptococcal infection. Streptococcal infections are generally spreading and may be severe. *Streptococcus pyogenes* produces a number of toxins. One of them, the streptolysin O, is an oxygen labile haemolysin and its presence is important in the diagnosis of recent streptococcal infection. In this situation patients have a raised level of antibodies to this streptolysin (raised Anti Streptolysin O or A S O, titre) (Fig. II,4). Practically all strains of *Streptococcus pyogenes* are sensitive to penicillin and erythromycin.

The delayed sequelae of streptococcal infection are rheumatic fever and acute glomerulonephritis.

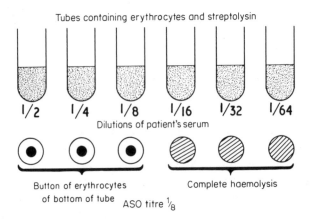

Tubes containing erythrocytes and streptolysin

1/2   1/4   1/8   1/16   1/32   1/64

Dilutions of patient's serum

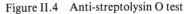

Button of erythrocytes of bottom of tube   Complete haemolysis

ASO titre 1/8

Figure II.4   Anti-streptolysin O test

Rheumatic fever is due to an immunological reaction to the primary streptococcal infection. There is a structural similarity between a protein antigen of the streptococcus and the myocardium and cross-reacting antibodies may be found. The precise mechanism of disease production is, however, not clear (Chapter X). Acute glomerulonephritis following streptococcal infection is also due to an immunological reaction the mechanisms of which again have not been elucidated (Chapter VI).

Group B Streptococci (Streptococcus agalactiae)

Beta haemolytic streptococci of Lancefield group B have recently been shown to be of importance as causes of meningitis and septicaemia in neonates (Chapter V).

Viridans streptococci

This is an α haemolytic streptococcus and a commensal in the mouth and upper respiratory tract. It is associated with an important disease, subacute bacterial endocarditis (Chapter X) and a member of this group has been considered to be a major contributor to tooth decay.

Streptococcus faecalis

This is also known as the enterococcus and is a commensal in the gut. It is often non-haemolytic, but β haemolytic strains occur and it is distinguished by its ability to grow on media containing bile salts, particularly MacConkey agar. It is a cause of urinary tract infection and subacute bacterial endocarditis.

Streptococcus pneumoniae (pneumococcus)

The pneumococcus is an α haemolytic diplococcus distinguished from *viridans streptococci* by its characteristic draughtsman colonies, sensitivity to optochin (diethylhydrocuprein) and bile solubility (Fig. II,5). Its polysaccharide capsule is important in pathogenicity, enabling the bacteria to resist phagocytosis. Many capsular types have been described and the distribution of these is important in preparing pneumococcal vaccines which are sometimes used prophylactically particularly following splenectomy. A commensal in the upper respiratory tract, a cause of lobar pneumonia and acute meningitis, it also plays a

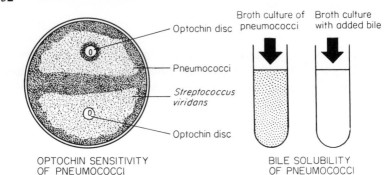

Figure II.5 Optochin sensitivity and bile solubility of pneumococci (Adapted from Gillies and Dodds: *Bacteriology Illustrated*, 4th Edition, by permission of Churchill Livingstone)

part in the exacerbations of chronic bronchitis and in some cases of bronchopneumonia. It is nearly always sensitive to penicillin.

Anaerobic streptococci

Commensal in the gut and the female genital tract, anaerobic streptococci are a cause of genital tract infection, particularly in the puerpuerium.

Gram-negative cocci

Neisseria

These are the most important Gram-negative cocci. The group includes two major pathogens *Neisseria gonorrhoeae* and *Neisseria meningitidis* and a number of commensals of the throat and upper respiratory tract including *Neisseria catarrhalis*.

Neisseria gonorrhoeae (gonococcus)

Gonococci are Gram-negative diplococci which require added CO_2 and heated blood agar for growth. They are distinguished from other neisseria by their biochemical reactions and their antigenic structure. This is demonstrated immunologically by the co-agglutination test and by immuno-fluorescent staining (Fig. II,6). Although originally sensitive to penicillin, penicillin resistant strains are now becoming increasingly common and this resistance may be mediated by β-lactamases (penicillinases). The organisms are the causative agent of gonorrhoea.

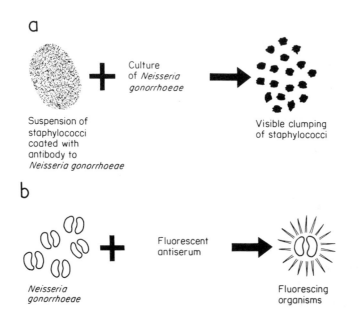

Figure II.6   Identification of *Neisseria gonorrhoeae*
a   co-agglutination   b   immunofluorescent test

Neisseria meningitidis (meningococcus)

This organism is indistinguishable microscopically from the gonococcus and requires similar cultural conditions. An occasional commensal in the upper respiratory tract, it is a causative agent of meningitis. Penicillin is the treatment of choice.

Gram-positive bacilli

These include three important genera, *Corynebacterium*, *Bacillus* and *Clostridium*. Listeria and erysipelothrix are less important human pathogens. Lactobacilli are commensals in the gut and the female genital tract and are non-pathogenic.

Corynebacteria

Corynebacteria are widely distributed as commensals in the upper respiratory tract and on the skin. These non-pathogenic strains are often referred to as diphtheroids. Anaerobic diphtheroids found on the skin are now included in the genus *Propionibacterium*. *Propionibacterium acnes* may be involved in the development of the lesions of the common skin disease acne. There is one important pathogen *Corynebacterium diphtheriae* but *Corynebacterium ulcerans* may occasionally cause a similar disease.

Corynebacterium diphtheriae

Characteristically the bacillus is rod shaped and contains metachromatic or volutin granules which may be demonstrated by Albert's stain. However, the classical appearance of the diphtheria bacillus described in the past is now rarely seen by many microbiologists due to the rarity of this disease in most developed countries. Selective media are used for the isolation of diphtheria bacilli; they include Loeffler's serum slope and tellurite agar on which the organism produces black colonies. There are three sub-groups, gravis, intermedius, and mitis which are distinguished by their biochemical reactions and colonial characteristics.

The main laboratory problem associated with *Corynebacterium diphtheriae* lies not in distinguishing this organism from commensal diphtheroids in the throat but in distinguishing pathogenic toxin-producers from the non-pathogenic non toxin-producing strains. Toxin production is mediated by a phage carried by some strains of the organism and toxin production may be demonstrated by an Elek plate or by guinea-pig inoculation (Figs. II,7 and II,8).

The important pathogenic effects are produced by the powerful entoxin acting on the heart, nervous system, and kidneys. The primary

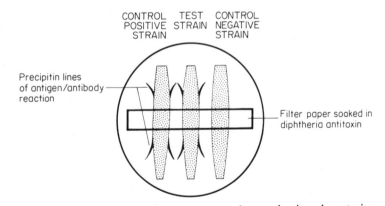

Figure II,7 Elek plate to demonstrate toxin production by strains of *Corynebacterium diphtheriae*

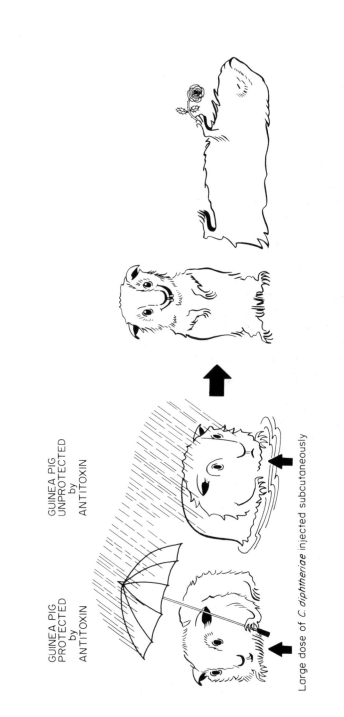

GUINEA PIG
PROTECTED
by
ANTITOXIN

GUINEA PIG
UNPROTECTED
by
ANTITOXIN

Large dose of *C. diphtheriae* injected subcutaneously

Figure II.8   Detection of toxin production by *Corynebacterium diphtheriae* using animal inoculation

lesion is often in the upper respiratory tract but the skin may be infected, particularly in warm climates.

The disease is uncommon in developed countries due to effective immunization.

Bacillus group

Members of the genus *Bacillus* are widely distributed in the environment, particularly in dirt, hay and soil. There are two pathogenic organisms, *Bacillus anthracis* and *Bacillus cereus*.

Bacillus anthracis

This is the causative agent of anthrax, a disease of herbivorous animals which spreads to man via hides, wool, and bone meal. The bacterium produces a spore which survives for long periods and enables dispersal of the organism to occur. The bacteria grow in long chains and produce colonies with the appearance of tangled hair. An unusual polypeptide capsule is produced. *Bacillus anthracis* can be distinguished from other aerobic spore bearing organisms which are widely distributed in the environment by its susceptibility to a specific phage.

Bacillus cereus

This causes a form of food poisoning due to the production of a toxin and is the only other human pathogen in the *Bacillus* genus.

Clostridia

Clostridia are widely distributed in the bowel of man and many animals and consequently are frequently found in the environment. They are all anaerobic spore bearing bacilli. There are three important human pathogens, *Clostridium perfringens*, *Clostridium tetani* and *Clostridium botulinum*. *Clostridium difficile* has in the last few years been recognized as a cause of pseudo-membranous colitis.

Clostridium perfringens (welchii)

This is a normal commensal of the bowel. *Cl. perfringens* is the common causative agent of gas gangrene and of the less destructive infection, anaerobic cellulitis. It is also the cause of a form of food poisoning.

Most strains are β haemolytic but some food poisoning strains are non-haemolytic.

The strains commonly associated with human disease produce an α toxin, a lecithinase. This produces an opacity on media containing lecithin due to the formation of an insoluble diglyceride. The reaction is inhibited by the specific toxin and the test, the Nagler test (Fig. II,9), is used in the identification of the organism.

Some other species of clostridia, including *Cl. oedematiens* and *Cl. septicum*, may be involved in anaerobic tissue infections.

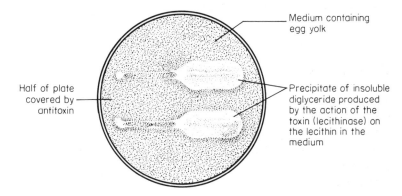

Medium containing egg yolk

Half of plate covered by antitoxin

Precipitate of insoluble diglyceride produced by the action of the toxin (lecithinase) on the lecithin in the medium

Figure II.9   Nagler plate to demonstrate the production of α toxin by *Clostridium perfringens* (Adapted from Gillies and Dodds: *Bacteriology Illustrated*, 4th Edition, by permission of Churchill Livingstone)

Clostridium tetani

This is the causative agent of tetanus. It is found in the gut of herbivorous animals and in some parts of the world in the gut of man. A strict anaerobe with a spherical terminal spore, it is motile producing a fine spreading growth. It produces an extremely powerful exotoxin, the tetanospasmin, which is responsible by its action on the nervous system for the production of the characteristic muscular spasms of the disease. The toxin is detected by its effect on mice; two groups of animals are used, one being protected by the specific antitoxin.

Clostridium botulinum

This is responsible for an uncommon form of food poisoning, botulism. It is a spore-forming anaerobe producing a powerful exotoxin which affects the parasympathetic nervous system.

Clostridium difficile

This organism has recently become of importance as a cause of pseudo-membranous colitis, a severe disease which can be a rare complication of antibiotic usage. It is an anaerobic spore-forming organism producing an exotoxin responsible for the illness. In the laboratory this exotoxin can be neutralized by antiserum prepared against the toxin of *Clostridium sordellii*, a related organism.

Listeria

Listeria monocytogenes

This is an aerobic, motile, Gram-positive bacillus, widely distributed in the animal population. It is a rare cause of meningitis and sometimes septicaemia in adults and of a generalized infection in infants.

Erysipelothrix

Erysipelothrix rhusiopathiae

This is a Gram-positive micro-aerophilic organism; predominantly an animal pathogen but occasionally causing skin infections in man.

Mycobacteria

These include *Mycobacterium tuberculosis* (human and bovine strains), *Mycobacterium leprae* and a number of other species which are often grouped together as the atypical mycobacteria.

Mycobacterium tuberculosis

This is the causative agent of tuberculosis. It is a slender, slightly curved rod. It is non-motile, non-sporing, non-capsulate, and a strict aerobe. There is a waxy substance in the cell wall which resists penetration with dyes. Once stained, however, it is difficult to remove the stain. This is the basis of the Ziehl–Neelsen staining method. Hot strong carbol fuchsin is used and decolorization is attempted with acid and alcohol. Methylene blue is added as the counterstain. Mycobacteria retain the carbol fuchsin and for this reason are often described as acid and alcohol fast bacilli.

Mycobacterium tuberculosis is a slow growing bacillus, colonies not appearing for at least 7–10 days, but up to 6–8 weeks may be required. Loewenstein–Jensen medium is often used to culture *M. tuberculosis*. It is a solidified egg medium which also contains malachite green. Liquid media may be used and Dubos medium is an example of one of these.

In the past guinea-pig inoculation was used to isolate *M. tuberculosis*. This is now seldom used except if necessary to prove virulence.

Mycobacterium tuberculosis occurs in two forms; the human strain *M. tuberculosis var hominis* and the bovine strain *M. tuberculosis var bovis*. These can be distinguished by their cultural characteristics.

Mycobacterium leprae

This is the causative agent of leprosy. *Mycobacterium leprae* organism is also acid and alcohol fast but cannot be cultured in artificial media. In laboratory animals it may be propagated in the foot pads of immunologically compromised mice and in armadillos.

Atypical mycobacteria

There are a number of atypical mycobacteria. All are acid and alcohol fast. *Mycobacterium marinum* is cultured at 30–33°C and is the causative agent of swimming pool granuloma. *Mycobacterium ulcerans* is a similar organism. It grows slowly on incubation at 32°C and is a cause of tropical skin ulcers. Other mycobacteria which less commonly cause human infection include *Mycobacterium kansasii* which is associated with lung disease.

Actinomyces and Nocardia

Actinomyces israelii

This is a non acid fast branching bacillus which grows in the form of a mycelium. It is anaerobic or micro-aerophilic and this can be nicely demonstrated by the use of shake culture (Fig. II,10). In pus, colonies are found which, because of their colour, are called sulphur granules. When crushed they show at the periphery radially arranged filaments with club shaped structures at the extremities. The filaments are Gram-positive but the clubs are Gram-negative.

Actinomyces israelii is the causative agent of actinomycosis, a chronic inflammatory condition often of the mouth (Chapter X).

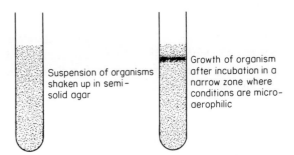

Suspension of organisms shaken up in semi-solid agar

Growth of organism after incubation in a narrow zone where conditions are micro-aerophilic

Figure II.10 Shake culture used to demonstrate that an organism is micro-aerophilic

Nocardia asteroides

This is also a branching filamentous organism but it is aerobic and acid fast. It may cause a disseminated infection characteristically with involvement of the central nervous system and also may be the causative agent of a mycetoma, Madura foot.

Gram-negative bacilli

These include: 1) members of the Enterobacteriaceae such as *Escherichia coli, Klebsiellae, Proteus, Shigellae,* and *Salmonellae*; 2) *Pseudomonas spp.*; 3) *Bacteroides*; 4) *Haemophilis influenzae*; 5) *Bordetella pertussis*; 6) *Yersinia pestis*; 7) *Brucella abortus, melitensis* and *suis*.

Enterobacteriaceae

All the members of this family are aerobic Gram-negative bacilli. They are distinguished by their biochemical reactions and then further subdivided by their antigenic structure.

Escherichia coli

This is a normal commensal of the large bowel of man and animals and is lactose fermenting. It can be subdivided by the use of antisera, to the O (somatic), H (flagellar), and K (capsular) antigens. Some strains may act as pathogens in the bowel of infants and less commonly of adults. It is the commonest cause of urinary tract infection and may also be associated with wound infections and neonatal meningitis.

Klebsiellae

Klebsiella strains are characterized by the production of a polysaccharide capsule which may be abundant and result in the formation of large mucoid or slimy colonies. The capsule is used to type the organism by means of the capsular swelling or 'quellung' reaction (Fig. II,11).

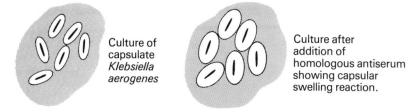

Culture of capsulate *Klebsiella aerogenes*

Culture after addition of homologous antiserum showing capsular swelling reaction.

Figure II.11   Capsular swelling or quellung reaction

Some species, particularly *Klebsiella pneumoniae*, are responsible for respiratory disease, particularly pneumonia. *Klebsiella aerogenes*, on the other hand, may be found in the large bowel and is an important cause of opportunistic infections elsewhere in the body.

Proteus

There are a number of species but as a group they are distinguished by their ability to swarm over the surface of an agar plate. Non-lactose fermenters, they are a cause of urinary tract infection and of a variety of other infections, generally low grade.

Shigellae

This group of organisms causes bacillary dysentery. There are four species, *Shigella dysenteriae*, *Shigella flexneri*, *Shigella boydii*, and *Shigella sonnei*. They can be distinguished by their biochemical reactions and antigenic structure. They are non lactose fermenting organisms, with the exception of *Shigella sonnei*, which is a late lactose fermenter, that is, it ferments lactose slowly. *Shigella sonnei* dysentery is common in the British Isles and in developed countries generally. The other organisms are of greater importance in tropical and sub-tropical countries.

Salmonellae

This enormous group may be divided into those organisms responsible for enteric fever, *Salmonella typhi* and *paratyphi* A, B, and C and the many hundreds of other salmonellas responsible for food poisoning. They are distinguished predominantly by their antigenic structure based on the O and H antigens and the possession by a few salmonellas including *Salmonella typhi* of a third antigen, a surface structure designated Vi.

The antigenic structure of the salmonellas is made more complex by the ability of the H antigens to exist in two separate phases with different antigenic expression. With rare exceptions the salmonellas do not ferment lactose.

Other Gram-negative bacilli

There are a large number of pseudomonads of which *Pseudomonas aeruginosa* is the most important human pathogen.

Pseudomonas aeruginosa

It is a free-living organism found in many moist situations and may, therefore, in hospitals be present in sinks, drains, and humidifiers.

It is also present in the bowel of a proportion of normal people. *Pseudomonas aeruginosa* is distinguished by the production of a green pigment and the possession of a characteristic sweetish smell. It does not ferment lactose. It is an opportunistic pathogen predominantly associated with urinary tract infection and serious intractable wound infection.

Bacteroides

These are strict anaerobes forming the predominant flora of the large bowel. The commonest species isolated from infections is *Bacteroides fragilis*. Bacteroides are now realized to be important pathogens in a variety of infections but particularly in wound infection following bowel surgery.

Haemophilus influenzae

This small cocco-bacillus is a causative agent of acute meningitis and of acute epiglottitis and is associated with exacerbations of chronic bronchitis. It is a fastidious organism, best cultured on heated blood agar. It requires two growth factors, haematin (X) and a co-enzyme (V). V factor is produced by staphylococci and the colonies of *Haemophilus influenzae* are larger when grown near staphylococci. This is satellitism (Fig. II,12). The organism may be capsulate, and capsular type b strains are particularly associated with meningitis.

There are a number of other *Haemophilus* spp. with different cultural requirements. *Haemophilus ducreyii* is the causative agent of chancroid, a venereal infection.

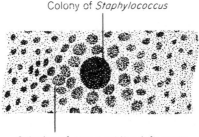

Figure II.12   Satellitism

Bordetella pertussis

This small Gram-negative cocco-bacillus is the causative agent of whooping cough. It requires an enriched medium for growth, and those usually used are charcoal agar or Bordet–Gengou, a potato glycerol agar medium. On this medium the small colonies have a metallic appearance.

Bordetella parapertussis is similar to *Bordetella pertussis* and may occasionally cause whooping cough but is antigenically distinct.

Yersinia

There are two human pathogens in this group.

Yersinia pestis

A short oval Gram-negative bacillus showing bipolar staining. It is the causative agent of plague (Chapter X).

Yersinia enterocolitica

This organism is a rare cause of enterocolitis and mesenteric lymphadentis in man.

Brucella

There are three species, *Brucella abortus*, *Brucella melitensis* and *Brucella suis* and all are aerobic cocco-bacilli. *Brucella abortus* requires additional CO_2 for isolation. They are slow growing and require enriched media for growth. The three species are differentiated by their CO_2 requirements, H_2S production, inhibition by dyes, and to a limited extent by their antigenic structure.

They are all causative agents of brucellosis (Chapter X).

Curved bacteria

Vibrios

Vibrios are widely distributed in the environment, and this group includes two human pathogens.

Vibrio cholerae

This is the causative agent of cholera. It is a curved, comma shaped bacillus and can be cultured at an alkaline pH; this property is made use of in its isolation. There are two strains, classical *Vibrio cholerae* and the El Tor strain. Both produce a potent enterotoxin which is responsible for the disease.

Vibrio parahaemolyticus

This marine vibrio causes food poisoning associated particularly with shellfish.

Campylobacter spp.

These organisms were previously classified with the vibrios. They are curved, micro-aerophilic, motile Gram-negative bacilli which are cultured at 43°C on special media. *Campylobacter jejuni* and *Campylobacter coli* are human pathogens causing a form of food poisoning.

Spirochaetes

These are spiral, motile, flexuous organisms. Their motility is due to bending and rotary movements and not due to the possession of flagella. There is a central contractile filament to which the body of the spirochaete is attached.

There are three groups of spirochaetes; *Leptospira*, *Treponema*, and *Borrelia*.

Leptospira

These have very fine regular spirals, are rapidly motile, and can be cultured in simple media. They are primarily pathogens of animals. *Leptospira icterohaemorrhagiae* is the causative agent of Weil's disease, while *Leptospira canicola* causes a milder illness in which meningitis is the main symptom.

Treponema

The spirals are less fine than those of the leptospira but are sharp and regular. *Treponema pallidum* is the causative agent of syphilis. It cannot be cultured on laboratory media.

Borrelia

These have loose, irregular spirals. *Borrelia vincentii* is found in the mouth and is associated with Vincent's angina. *Borrelia recurrentis* and *Borrelia duttoni* may be cultured anaerobically in blood-containing media. They are the causative agents of relapsing fever.

Mycoplasmas

These are bacteria and can be grown on cell-free media where they produce a characteristic 'fried egg' colony. However, they have no cell wall, and are pleomorphic and highly fragile. The most important human pathogen is *Mycoplasma pneumoniae*, a causative agent of pneumonia. They may be distinguished from L forms of bacteria which also produce no cell wall because L forms will revert to a normal bacterial form, but mycoplasmas will not. L forms are non-pathogenic.

The organisms previously designated T strain mycoplasmas, which are associated with urethritis, are now called *Ureaplasma urealyticum*.

Rickettsiae

These are also bacteria but are obligate, intracellular parasites. They are Gram-negative, pleomorphic, non-motile organisms. They occur in the alimentary tract of arthropods, and in man they cause a variety of forms of typhus, which may be spread by lice, fleas, ticks or mites.

Coxiella burnetti

Although resembling the rickettsiae in being an obligate, intracellular parasite, this organism has a number of properties which distinguish it. It is the causative agent of Q (query) fever.

VIRUSES

These may be divided into DNA and RNA viruses. Those which cause human disease, with their major characteristics, are listed below. (Fig. II,13).

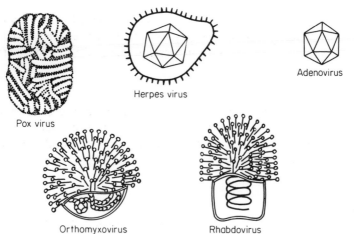

Pox virus

Herpes virus

Adenovirus

Orthomyxovirus

Rhabdovirus

Figure II.13　The structure of some viruses (Adapted in part from Cruikshank: *Medical Microbiology*, 12th Edition, by permission of Churchill Livingstone)

DNA Viruses

These include pox-viruses, herpesviruses, adenoviruses and papovaviruses.

Pox-viruses

Smallpox, cowpox and vaccinia (used for vaccination) are pox-viruses.

They are large brick-shaped viruses which produce pocks on the chorio-allantoic membrane of the chick. Orf virus is also a member of this group.

Herpesvirus

Herpes simplex, varicella-zoster, cytomegalovirus, and Epstein-Barr virus are herpesviruses. They all form icosahedral particles.

Herpes simplex virus

There are two types of *Herpes simplex* virus. Type 1 causes skin lesions, usually on the face, herpes febrilis or 'cold sores'. Type 2 is particularly responsible for genital lesions. Both types can be grown in tissue culture and both produce pocks on the chorioallantoic membrane of the fertile hen's egg.

Varicella-zoster virus

Varicella-zoster is one virus which has two clinical manifestations, chicken pox and shingles. Shingles (zoster) is due to reactivation of dormant virus. The virus can be grown in human cells in tissue culture.

Cytomegalovirus

Cytomegalovirus is so called because affected cells are large. They also contain intra-nuclear inclusions, 'owls' eyes'. These are seen in tissue cultures of the virus. It is an opportunistic pathogen and may cause severe congenital infections.

Epstein-Barr virus

Epstein-Barr virus is associated with the tumours of Burkitt's lymphoma and is the cause of many cases of infectious mononucleosis (glandular fever).

Adenoviruses

There are 33 serological types of adenoviruses. They form icosahedral particles with fibres projecting from the vertices. They grow slowly in tissue culture and are responsible for a variety of infections particularly of the upper respiratory tract and conjunctiva.

Papovaviruses

These are DNA tumour viruses forming small icosahedral particles. They include papilloma virus, which is associated with human warts, a number of viruses associated with tumours in animals, and the virus of a rare human disease, progressive multifocal leucoencephalopathy.

RNA viruses

These include orthomyxoviruses, paramyxoviruses, rhabdoviruses, picornaviruses, reoviruses, togaviruses, and arenoviruses.

Orthomyxoviruses

These are the causative agents of influenza. They consist of helically coiled ribonucleoprotein surrounded by an envelope with projections of haemagglutinin and neuraminidase. Influenza A causes epidemics of infection, while influenza B is associated mainly with sporadic disease. These viruses can be cultured in monkey kidney tissue culture.

One of the most important attributes of the influenza virus is its ability to undergo antigenic change. This may be major (antigenic shift) or minor (antigenic drift).

Antigenic shift is associated with the possession of a new haemagglutinin or neuraminidase, or both. These changes may arise as a result of recombination with avian or animal strains of influenza virus. Antigenic drift is a much smaller change in the haemagglutinin and is due to mutation. The major antigenic changes are significant because they enable the virus to spread in a community which lacks immunity to the new influenza strain. It also makes it difficult to produce a satisfactory vaccine.

Paramyxoviruses

These are in many ways similar to the orthomyxoviruses. They possess helical symmetry, haemagglutinate, and grow in monkey kidney tissue cultures. They include parainfluenza virus which causes colds, respiratory tract infections and croup, mumps virus and measles virus.

Rhabdoviruses

The most important of these is the rabies virus which contains helically coiled nucleoprotein and is bullet shaped. It can be grown in tissue culture. Marburg virus is associated with African green monkeys and has only occasionally spread to man. The virus can be grown in tissue culture and the particles are unusual in that they are filamentous.

Picornaviruses

These form icosahedral particles and they include the enteroviruses and rhinoviruses. The enteroviruses are so called because they are associated with the alimentary tract, but nevertheless they all cause disease of the central nervous system. They include polio viruses, coxsackie viruses and echo viruses. Most will grow in tissue culture. Coxsackie viruses are distinguished by their pathogenicity for suckling mice. Rhinoviruses cause the common cold. They are similar to the enteroviruses but are distinguished by their inactivation at acid pH and growth in tissue culture at 33°C rather than at 37°C.

Reoviruses

The most important of these are the rotaviruses, so called because of their typical wheel-like appearance on electron microscopy. They are a cause of diarrhoea, particularly in young children and infants. Although rotaviruses are classified as reoviruses, there are differences between them and the typical reoviruses, which are of doubtful pathogenicity for man.

Togaviruses

These form particles with icosahedral symmetry and can be grown in tissue culture. Most are spread by arthropods and cause encephalitis and haemorrhagic fever. Yellow fever is an important disease caused by a togavirus.

Rubella is caused by a virus which is provisionally classified as a non-arthropod-borne togavirus. It exhibits helical symmetry and haem-agglutinates chick red cells.

Arenaviruses

These viruses are characterized by the presence of internal granules and they can be grown in tissue culture. Lymphocytic choriomeningitis is caused by an arenavirus and so is Lassa fever, a more severe disease.

FUNGI

The fungi of medical importance can be most easily considered in three groups: candida, the dermatophytes, and the fungi associated with systemic infections (Fig. II,14).

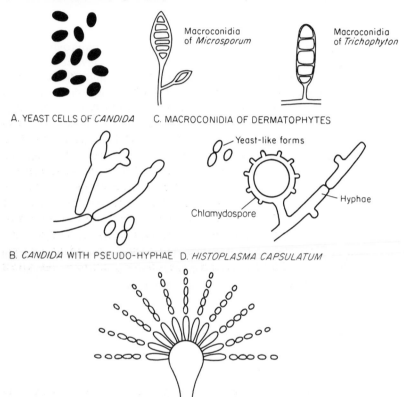

A. YEAST CELLS OF *CANDIDA*

Macroconidia of *Microsporum*

Macroconidia of *Trichophyton*

C. MACROCONIDIA OF DERMATOPHYTES

Yeast-like forms

Hyphae

Chlamydospore

B. *CANDIDA* WITH PSEUDO-HYPHAE D. *HISTOPLASMA CAPSULATUM*

E. CONIDIOPHORE OF *ASPERGILLUS FUMIGATUS*

Figure II.14   Fungi

Candida spp.

These form oval, Gram-positive yeast cells. Pseudo-hyphae may be seen invading cells when the fungus is acting as a pathogen. Candida can be cultured on ordinary laboratory media. *Candida albicans* is the most common human pathogen but other candida species may also be pathogenic.

Candida albicans is distinguished by its ability to form germ tubes in human serum, and by the formation of characteristic chlamydospores when inoculated into corn-meal agar (Fig. II,14).

The most common infections are superficial infections of the mouth and of the vagina and vulva, but systemic infections also occur.

Dermatophytes

These cause tinea, a superficial infection of the skin, hair or nails. Three genera are involved, *Trichophyton, Epidermophyton* and *Microsporum*, which may be distinguished by their characteristic macroconidia (Fig. II,14). The diagnosis is made by the examination of skin scrapings, nail clippings or hair. These are treated with 30% KOH and gently warmed. This dissolves the cells and the fungal hyphae can be seen. The fungi can be cultivated on Sabouraud's medium; after 1–3 weeks the characteristic fungal colonies appear. Species identification is made on the macroscopic appearance of the colony and microscopically. Some common examples of fungal species are *Trichophyton rubrum* which causes infections of the nails and the skin of the feet. *Trichophyton mentagrophytes* can attack the scalp, hair, skin, and nails. *Microsporum audouini* causes scalp ringworm in children and *Epidermophyton floccosum* can affect the skin of the groin.

Fungi associated with systemic infections

Cryptococcus neoformans

This is a rare cause of meningitis. The organism is widely distributed in the soil and in birds and animals. The yeasts can be distinguished in the cerebrospinal fluid (CSF) by the presence of large capsules and they can be cultured on Sabouraud's agar.

Blastomycosis dermatitidis

This causes a chronic granulomatosis condition of the skin and it may also involve the lungs with generalized spread. It is seen in North America and the source of the infection may be the soil. The disease is diagnosed by culture of the dimorphic fungus on blood agar or Sabouraud's agar.

Blastomycosis brasiliensis

This is the cause of a similar condition occurring in South America.

Histoplasma capsulatum

This also is a dimorphic fungus and is the cause of histoplasmosis which may be manifest as a chronic systemic granulomatous disease or as a benign lesion localized to the lung. The disease is most commonly seen in the Mississippi valley, where the organism is found in the soil. *Histoplasma capsulatum* can be cultured on blood agar or Sabouraud's agar.

Coccidioides immitis

This is a dimorphic fungus causing coccidiomycosis, a generalized granulomatous infection which is usually benign. It is generally confined to the Northwest USA. This fungus also can be cultured on blood agar and Sabouraud's agar.

Aspergillus fumigatus

This is a saprophytic fungus. On culture it produces greenish coloured colonies. It is recognized by the characteristic conidiophores (Fig. II,14). It may act as a pathogen in previously damaged lung where it typically forms a giant colony, an aspergilloma.

PROTOZOA

Protozoa are unicellular eucaryocytic organisms and a number of them are human pathogens. The organisms and the diseases they cause in man are discussed in more detail in later chapters.

Rhizopoda

These are protozoa with pseudopodia.

Entamoeba histolytica

This is an important member of this group (Chapter VIII) and is the causative agent of amoebic dysentery and liver abscess in man. Transmission of the disease from man to man occurs via ingestion of the

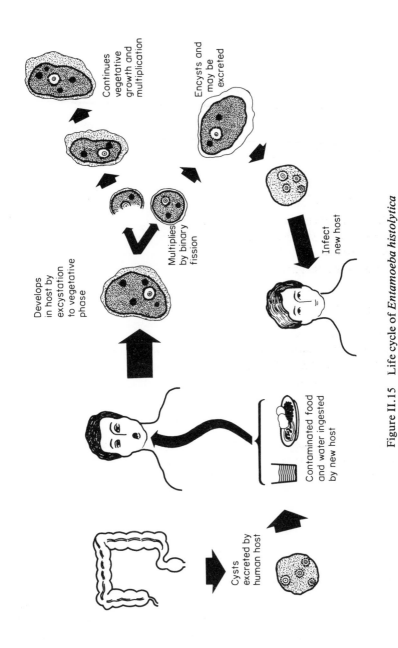

Figure II.15   Life cycle of *Entamoeba histolytica*

encysted form in water and food contaminated by human excreta. The life cycle of *Entamoeba histolytica* is shown in Fig. II,15.

Mastigophora

These are protozoa with flagella. The most important of the Mastigophora are the haemoflagellates, the trypanosomes (Chapter XIII). Other important Mastigophora are *Trichomonas vaginalis* and *Giardia lamblia*. *Trichomonas vaginalis* is a common cause of vaginitis and vaginal discharge (Chapter VII). The diagnosis is made by demonstrating the presence of the characteristic trophozoites. Treatment is by metronidazole. *Giardia lamblia* is sometimes found in the duodenum and the upper ileum of man where it may cause malabsorption and diarrhoea. Diagnosis is made by demonstrating the presence of the trophozoites or cysts (Fig. I,6) and duodenal intubation may be necessary to do this. Metronidazole is useful in this condition also.

Sporozoa

These protozoa do not have any special organs of locomotion. The important pathogens are the plasmodia, the causative agent of malaria (Chapter XIII).

Ciliata

The only human pathogen which is a ciliated protozoon is *Balantidium coli*. The pig is the reservoir of infection but the organism may give rise to dysentery in man. It is much less commonly seen than amoebic dysentery.

Protozoa of uncertain classification

Toxoplasma gondii

This protozoon is the cause of widespread infection, usually sub-clinical. It can, however, cause serious damage to the foetus if contracted by the mother during pregnancy (Chapter XIII).

Pneumocystis carinii

The status of this organism is uncertain. It is probably a protozoon and is an important cause of pneumonia in immunocompromised individuals. Diagnosis is made by biopsy. Treatment is by cotrimoxazole in high dosage, or pentamidine.

MAJOR MICRO-ORGANISMS OF MEDICAL IMPORTANCE

Names	Characteristics	Normal Habitat	Diseases Caused
	BACTERIA		
	Gram-positive cocci		
Staphylococcus aureus *Staphylococcus pyogenes*	Golden colonies. Arranged in clusters. Coagulase, phosphatase and DNAase positive.	Anterior nares and skin of some normal individuals.	Boils, carbuncles, whitlows, wound infections. Food poisoning.
Staphylococcus albus *Staphylococcus epidermidis*	White colonies.	Normal skin.	Sub-acute bacterial endocarditis.
Streptococcus pyogenes (Group A streptococci)	β haemolytic. Arranged in chains. Lancefield group A	Anterior nares and throat of some normal individuals	Tonsillitis, scarlet fever, erysipelas, and wound infections. Delayed sequelae are rheumatic fever and glomerulo-nephritis.
Streptococcus agalactiae (Group B streptococci)	β haemolytic.	Genital tract of some normal individuals.	Meningitis and septicaemia in neonates.
Streptococcus viridans	α haemolytic.	Mouth and throat.	Sub-acute bacterial endocarditis.
Streptococcus faecalis Enterococcus (Group D streptococci)	Can be cultured on media containing bile salts.	Bowel of man.	Urinary tract infection. Sub-acute bacterial endocarditis.
Streptococcus pneumoniae Pneumococcus	α haemolytic draughtsman colonies. Bile soluble, optochin sensitive, capsulated diplococcus.	Upper respiratory tract of some normal individuals.	Lobar pneumonia. Meningitis.

Names	Characteristics	Normal Habitat	Diseases caused
Anaerobic streptococci	Strict anaerobes.	Bowel and female genital tract.	Wound infections and infections of genital tract.
Gram-negative cocci			
Neisseria gonorrhoeae Gonococcus	Gram-negative intracellular diplococci. Require heated blood agar and added CO_2 for growth	Genital tract of infected persons.	Gonorrhoea.
Neisseria meningitidis Meningococcus	As gonococcus	Upper respiratory tract of some normal people.	Meningococcal meningitis.
Gram-positive bacilli			
Corynebacterium diphtheriae gravis, intermedius, and mitis	Contain metachromatic or volutin granules. Pathogenic strains are toxin producers.	Upper respiratory tract of some normal people.	Diphtheria.
Bacillus anthracis	Spore-bearing. Forms a colony with the appearance of tangled hair.	Bowel of herbivores.	Anthrax.
Bacillus cereus	Spore bearing.	Widely distributed in the environment.	Food poisoning.
Clostridium perfringens *Clostridium welchii*	Anaerobic. Spore bearing. β haemolytic.	Bowel of man and animals.	Gas gangrene. Food poisoning.
Clostridium tetani	Anaerobic. Terminal spore. Fine spreading, growth. Powerful exotoxin produced by pathogenic strains	Gut of herbivorous animals.	Tetanus.
Clostridium botulinum	Anaerobic. Spore bearing. Powerful exotoxin produced.	Soil. Marine sediment.	Botulism.

Names	Characteristics	Normal Habitat	Diseases Caused
Clostridium difficile	Anaerobic. Spore bearing. Exotoxin produced.	Not known — possibly human gut	Pseudo-membranous colitis.
Listeria monocytogenes	Aerobic. Motile.	Widely distributed in animal population.	Meningitis and septicaemia
Erysipelothrix rhusiopathiae	Micro-aerophilic.	Widely distributed in animal population.	Skin infections.

Mycobacteria

Names	Characteristics	Normal Habitat	Diseases Caused
Mycobacterium tuberculosis var hominis var bovis	Acid and alcohol fast. Slow growing.	var hominis; infected individuals. var bovis; infected cattle.	Tuberculosis.
Mycobacterium leprae	Acid and alcohol fast. Cannot be cultured in artificial media.	Infected individuals.	Leprosy.
Mycobacterium marinum	Cultured at 30–33°C	Swimming pools. Fish tanks.	Swimming pool granuloma.
Mycobacterium ulcerans	Cultured at 32°C	Infected individuals.	Tropical skin ulcers. Buruli ulcer.
Mycobacterium kansasii	Acid and alcohol fast. Pigments in the light.	Infected individuals	Pulmonary disease similar to tuberculosis.

Higher bacteria

Names	Characteristics	Normal Habitat	Diseases Caused
Actinomyces israelii	Anaerobic or micro-aerophilic. Branching filaments.	Mouth of some normal individuals.	Actinomycosis.
Nocardia madurae	Aerobic. Acid fast branching filaments.	Infected individuals. Soil.	Madura foot.

Names	Characteristics	Normal Habitat	Diseases Caused
Gram-negative bacilli			
Escherichia coli	Lactose fermenting. Can be cultured on media containing bile salts.	Bowel of man and animals.	Urinary tract and wound infections. Septicaemia. Meningitis. Gastro-enteritis in infants. Traveller's diarrhoea.
Klebsiella pneumoniae	Lactose fermenting coliform. Capsulate.	Upper respiratory tract.	Pneumonia.
Klebsiella aerogenes	Lactose fermenting coliform. Capsulate.	Bowel of man and animals.	Opportunistic infections particularly of urinary tract.
Proteus spp.	Non-lactose fermenters. Swarming growth of some species.	Bowel of man and animals.	A variety of low grade infections particularly of the urinary tract.
Shigella dysenteriae, flexneri, boydii, sonnei	Non-lactose fermenters except sonnei which is a late lactose fermenter.	Bowel of infected individuals and some normal people.	Bacillary dysentery.
Salmonella typhi and *paratyphi* A, B, and C	Non-lactose fermenters.	Bowel of infected patients and some normal individuals.	Enteric fever.
Salmonella typhimurium and many other salmonellas	Non-lactose fermenters.	Bowel of animals, infected patients and some normal individuals.	Food poisoning.
Pseudomonas aeruginosa (pyocyanea)	Non-lactose fermenter. Produces a characteristic green pigment.	Free living, found in ponds, streams, sinks, and drains, and in the bowel of some normal individuals.	A variety of low grade infections particularly of burns and of the urinary tract.

Names	Characteristics	Normal Habitat	Diseases Caused
Bacteroides fragilis	Strict anaerobes.	Bowel of man and animals.	Many infections but particularly wound infections following bowel surgery.
Haemophilus influenzae	Requires two growth factors X and V. Capsulate.	Upper respiratory tract of normal individuals.	Meningitis. Epiglottitis. Exacerbations of chronic bronchitis.
Bordetella pertussis	Enriched medium required for growth.	Respiratory tract of infected individuals.	Whooping cough.
Yersinia pestis	Bipolar staining.	Rats.	Plague.
Brucella abortus melitensis and *suis*	Slow growing cocco-bacilli	Cows, sheep and pigs.	Brucellosis.
Curved bacteria			
Vibrio cholerae and El Tor strain	Comma shaped. Cultured at alkaline pH. Produce an enterotoxin.	Bowel of infected individuals.	Cholera.
Vibrio parahaemolyticus	Comma shaped bacillus.	Sea water.	Food poisoning.
Campylobacter jejuni and *Campylobacter coli*	Curved; Micro-aerophilic. Cultured at 43°C	Widely distributed in the bowel of domestic animals.	Food poisoning.
Spirochaetes			
Leptospira icterohaem-orrhagiae and *L. canicola*	Spirochaetes with fine regular spirals.	Widely distributed in animals, particularly rats (ictero-haemorrhagiae) and dogs (canicola).	Leptospirosis.
Treponema pallidum	Spirochaete with sharp, regular spirals.	Infected individuals.	Syphilis.

Names	Characteristics	Normal Habitat	Diseases Caused
Borrelia vincentii	Spirochaete with loose irregular spirals.	Normal mouth.	Vincent's angina.
Borrelia recurrentis and *Borrelias duttonii*	Spirochaetes with loose irregular spirals	Lice (*recurrentis*). Ticks (*duttonii*). Small rodents. Infected individuals.	Relapsing fever.
Mycoplasmas			
Mycoplasma pneumoniae	No cell wall; Pleomorphic; Characteristic 'fried egg' colonies.	Infected individuals.	Pneumonia.
Ureaplasma urealyticum (T strain mycoplasma)	No cell wall. Pleomorphic.	Infected individuals.	Urethritis.
Rickettsiae			
Rickettsia prowazekii	Obligate intracellular parasite.	Lice. Infected individuals.	Typhus.
Rickettsia rickettsii	Obligate intracellular parasite.	Ticks. Small mammals. Infected individuals.	Rocky Mountain Spotted Fever
Rickettsia tsutsugamushi	Obligate intracellular parasite.	Mites. Small rodents. Infected individuals.	Scrub typhus.
Rickettsia quintana	The only rickettsia that is not an obligate intracellular parasite.	Lice. Infected individuals.	Trench fever.
Coxiella burnetti	Not now classified as a rickettsia An obligate intracellular parasite.	Ticks. Small wild mammals. Sheep and cattle.	Q (query) fever.

Names	Characteristics	Normal Habitat	Diseases Caused
	VIRUSES		
	DNA viruses		
	Pox-viruses		
Variola major	Large brick shaped virus.	Infected individuals.	Smallpox. (now eradicated)
Vaccinia	Morphologically similar to variola.	None.	Used to vaccinate against smallpox.
Orf	Characteristic entwined appearance.	Infected sheep.	Contagious pustular dermatitis (of sheep) Orf (of man)
	Herpesviruses		
Herpes simplex 1 and 2	Large icosahedral virus. Can be grown in tissue culture and on chorio-alantoic membrane.	Infected individuals in whom infection may be latent.	Herpes febrilis or cold sores (type 1) Genital lesions (type 2)
Varicella zoster virus	Similar to other members of this group.	Infected individuals in whom infection may be latent.	Chicken pox. Shingles.
Cytomegalovirus	Similar to other members of this group. Causes enlargement of infected cells and intra-nuclear inclusions 'owls' eyes'.	Infected individuals.	Opportunistic and congenital infections.
Epstein-Barr virus	Morphologically identical to Herpes simplex virus.	Infected individuals.	Associated with Burkitt's lymphoma Many cases of infectious mononucleosis (glandular fever)
Adenoviruses	Icosahedral particles with fibres projecting from vertices. 33 serological types.	Infected individuals.	Infections of upper respiratory tract Conjunctivitis

Names	Characteristics	Normal Habitat	Diseases Caused
Papovaviruses	Tumour viruses	Infected individuals.	Warts in man. Tumours in animals.

RNA viruses

Orthomyxoviruses

Names	Characteristics	Normal Habitat	Diseases Caused
Influenza A and B	Helically coiled ribonucleoprotein with an envelope with projections of haemagglutinin and neuraminidase. Undergoes major and minor antigenic changes	Infected individuals.	Influenza.

Paramyxoviruses

Names	Characteristics	Normal Habitat	Diseases Caused
Parainfluenza virus Mumps virus Measles virus	Helical symmetry. Haemagglutinate. Grow in monkey kidney tissue culture.	Infected individuals.	Colds. Upper respiratory tract infections and (parainfluenza virus). Mumps. Measles.

Rhabdoviruses

Names	Characteristics	Normal Habitat	Diseases Caused
Rabies virus	Helically coiled ribonucleoprotein. Bullet shaped.	Infected animals dogs, foxes, jackals, wolves, etc.	Rabies.
Marburg virus	Filamentous particles.	African green monkeys.	Marburg disease.

Picornoviruses

Names	Characteristics	Normal Habitat	Diseases Caused
Enteroviruses Polio virus Coxsackie A and B viruses.	Icosahedral particles.	Alimentary tract of man.	Polio (polio virus). Meningitis (Coxsackie A virus). Bornholm disease (Coxsackie B virus). Fever, Meningitis.
Echovirus Rhinoviruses	Growth occurs at 33°C not 37°C	Infected individuals.	Common cold.
Rotavirus	Typical wheel-like appearance.	Infected individuals and carriers.	Diarrhoea, particularly in infants.

Names	Characteristics	Normal Habitat	Diseases Caused
Togaviruses	Icosahedral particles. Spread by arthropods.	Animal reservoir particularly monkeys.	Encephalitis and haemorrhagic fevers Yellow fever
Rubella virus	Non-arthropod-borne togavirus	Infected individuals	German measles (Rubella)
Arenaviruses			
Lymphocytic chorio-meningitis virus	Internal granules	Small rodents	Benign lymphocytic chorio-meningitis
Lassa fever virus		Infected individuals	Lassa fever.
Fungi			
Candida albicans	Yeast. Forms germ tubes in human serum and chlamydospores in corn meal agar	Infected individuals and carriers	Superficial infections particularly of mouth and vagina
Dermatophytes			
Trichophyton, Microsporum, and Epidermophyton spp.	Fungal hyphae can be seen in infected skin. Characteristic macroconidia are formed	Infected individuals, animals, and the environment.	Tinea of hair, skin, and nails
Cryptococcus neoformans	Yeasts with a large capsule	Widely distributed in birds, animals, and soil	Cryptococcosis. Meningitis
Blastomyces dermatitidis and *brasiliensis*	Dimorphic fungus	Present in soil	Blastomycosis, a chronic granulomatous condition of the skin.
Histoplasma capsulatum	Dimorphic fungus	Present in soil, particularly in the Mississippi valley	Histoplasmosis, a benign lesion of lung or a chronic systemic disease
Coccidioides immitis	Dimorphic fungus	Soil, rodents and domestic animals	Coccidiomycosis, a generalized benign infection

Names	Characteristics	Normal Habitat	Diseases Caused
Aspergillus fumigatus	Greenish colonies with characteristic conidiophores	Widely distributed in the environment	Aspergilloma in previously damaged lung

PROTOZOA

Rhizopoda

Entamoeba Histolytica	Amoeba with a cystic form.	Infected individuals and carriers	Amoebic dysentery Hepatic abscess

Mastigophora

Trichomonas vaginalis	Flagellated protozoa	Infected individuals and carriers	Vaginitis
Giardia lamblia	Flagellated protozoa	Infected individuals	Intestinal giardiasis Malabsorption Diarrhoea
Trypanosome gambiense and *rhodesiense*	Haemoflagellates	Man. Antelope (rhodesiense)	Sleeping sickness
Trypanosome cruzi	Haemoflagellates	Man. Armadillo	Chaga's disease South American trypanasomiasis
Leishmania donovani	Haemoflagellates	Man, dogs, jackals, gerbils, etc.	Kala-azar. Cutaneous leishmaniasis

Sporozoa

Plasmodium vivax falciparum malariae ovale	Complex life cycle in man and anopheline mosquito. Characteristic morphology of individual species can be seen on examination of blood of infected individual	Infected individuals	Malaria

Ciliata

Balantidium coli	Ciliated protozoa with cystic phase	Pig	Dysentery

Names	Characteristics	Normal Habitat	Diseases Caused
	Unclassified protozoa		
Pneumocystis carinii	Probably a protozoan but even this is doubtful	Man	Pneumonia in immuno-compromised individuals
Toxoplasma gondii	A protozoan of uncertain classification	Man and many animals including cats and dogs	Congenital toxoplasmosis Toxoplasmosis usually in immuno-compromised individuals

CHAPTER III

Infections of the
Upper Respiratory Tract

These include the common cold, sinusitis, sore throats, laryngitis, epiglottitis, tracheitis, and diphtheria.

COMMON COLD

The common cold is probably the most frequent malady suffered by man. It is a mild illness with rhinorrhoea, sore and sometimes slightly inflamed throat and a low grade pyrexia. It is caused by any one of a number of viruses, most commonly rhinovirus, corona virus, and adenovirus spread from person to person by droplet and aerosol. The number of possible infectious agents and their antigenic variation mean that natural immunity is not acquired to any extent and immunization is not a practical proposition. Only symptomatic treatment is necessary although antibiotics may have to be used to treat secondary bacterial infections if these should follow.

SINUSITIS

This usually arises due to secondary bacterial invasion following a primary viral infection. Acute infections often follow the common cold and there may be pain, nasal discharge and fever. Occasionally severe pain may be experienced. Chronic sinusitus may follow repeated acute attacks. The bacteria commonly isolated from sinusitis are *Streptococcus pneumoniae*, *Haemophilus influenzae* and *Staphylococcus aureus*. Antibiotics may be used in treatment but the promotion of good drainage from the affected sinuses is probably more valuable.

SORE THROAT

Sore throats may vary from a mild illness requiring little treatment to a severe tonsillitis with spread to local lymph glands and to the middle ear.

Streptococcus pyogenes is the most important pathogen but often the causative agent is viral, enteroviruses and adenoviruses being most frequently found. Especially in young adults the possibility of glandular fever should be considered (see below).

Treatment of streptococcal sore throat should be with penicillin or erythromycin. Although most sore throats, particularly in children, are treated without a definitive microbiological diagnosis being made, this can be of value and throat swabs may be taken, plated on to blood agar medium and the characteristic colonies of *Streptococcus pyogenes* seen surrounded by a clear zone of β haemolysis. The importance of streptococcal infection lies in the very serious sequelae which may occur. These are acute rheumatic fever (Chapter X) or acute glomerulo-nephritis (Chapter VI) which may arise 10–20 days after the initial infection. They are much less commonly seen now than they were previously, probably due to the ready use of antibiotics in the treatment of sore throat. No treatment other than symptomatic is required for viral sore throat.

INFECTIOUS MONONUCLEOSIS (GLANDULAR FEVER)

Although in many respects a generalized infection, this disease is considered in this chapter because it most often presents primarily as a sore throat accompanied by lymphadenopathy. There may also be a rash, and the spleen and liver may be affected. The causative organism is a herpes virus, the Epstein-Barr virus (EBV) which is commonly found in the saliva, and the disease is spread from person to person. The onset of disease follows an incubation period of 4–6 weeks, and symptoms can be very variable. The disease can be quite debilitating and relapses may occur over several months to 1 or 2 years.

Laboratory diagnosis is by the demonstration of abnormal mononuclear cells in the peripheral blood and by the Paul Bunnell test. This test depends on the demonstration in the patient's serum of antibodies which agglutinate sheep red cells. This type of antibody reacting with some unrelated material not its specific antigen is known as a heterophil antibody. The antibody can be further characterized by its titre in the test being reduced following absorption by ox red blood cells but not by guinea-pig kidney cell emulsion. Diagnosis is not generally made by virus isolation, but serum antibodies to EBV can be demonstrated by immuno-fluorescence techniques with infected tissue cell lines. The presence of IgM antibodies indicates recent infection. There is no specific treatment but recovery is practically always complete.

LARYNGITIS, TRACHEITIS, AND EPIGLOTTITIS

All these conditions are generally viral; para-influenza viruses are common. However, acute epiglottitis in children which may be a severe disease is due to *Haemophilus influenzae* type b and requires treatment with ampicillin.

DIPHTHERIA

Diphtheria is now uncommon in developed countries due to successful immunization programmes. The disease is due to the effects of the potent exotoxin produced by the organism *Corynebacterium diphtheriae*. The exotoxin produces systemic effects, particularly myocardial damage. The primary lesion is often in the throat where the characteristic 'false membrane' is found, but skin diphtheria is not uncommon particularly in warm climates. Toxin production is phage mediated and non-toxigenic *Corynebacterium diphtheriae* strains are frequent.

Immunization against the disease is achieved by the use of toxoid. Immunity to the disease may be examined for by the Schick test, in which small amounts of toxin are injected intradermally. In a non-immune individual an area of reddening is produced. The Schick test is now less frequently used than previously and levels of circulating anti-toxin may be measured.

Diagnosis of diphtheria must be made clinically as it is essential to administer anti-toxin as quickly as possible. The diagnosis may be confirmed in the laboratory by isolation of *Corynebacterium diphtheriae* on a Loeffler's serum slope or on tellurite medium. Gravis, intermedius and mitis strains may be differentiated biochemically but the important property of the organism is toxin production. This is now usually examined for by use of an Elek plate (fig. II, 7) on which precipitin lines due to the reaction of the toxin produced by the organism with antitoxin can be seen. Toxin production may also be looked for by using anti-toxin protected and unprotected animals, usually guinea-pigs. According to the particular test used the indicator of toxin production may be the development of a skin lesion or may be death of the unprotected animal.

Treatment of the disease is by large doses of anti-toxin, and penicillin or erythromycin is given. Symptomless carriers are treated by erythromycin and it is now becoming customary to treat carriers of non-toxigenic strains also. *Corynebacterium ulcerans* may also be toxigenic and produce a similar but generally milder disease.

INFECTIONS OF THE EAR

Infections of the middle ear (otitis media) usually arise by spread of organisms from the throat via the Eustachian tube. *Streptococcus pneumoniae*, *Haemophilus influenzae*, and *Streptococcus pyogenes* are organisms most commonly involved. There is pyrexia and pain in the ear which may be severe. The tympanic membrane will be involved and it may rupture and pus will then be discharged through the external auditory meatus. This is a serious infection, as repeated attacks of otitis media result in impaired hearing, and antibiotic therapy should be started as soon as possible after a throat swab has been taken to determine the causative agent.

Untreated otitis media may spread locally to give rise to mastoiditis, an infection of the mastoid process which may need surgical treatment. Intracranial spread is also a possibility. Fortunately due to effective antibiotic therapy these complications are now seldom seen.

Otitis externa is an inflammation of the external auditory meatus. It is common and is usually low grade. A whole variety of organisms may be associated with the disease. These may be bacterial or fungal and include such organisms as *Proteus mirablis*, *Pseudomonas aeruginosa*, and *Aspergillis fumigatus*. Topical antibiotic therapy is required.

INFECTIONS OF THE EYE

These include styes, conjunctivitis, and deeper infections, such as keratitis and endophthalmitis.

Styes

Styes are infections associated with the root of an eye-lash and are small localized collections of pus. Most are mild and self-limiting, and antibiotic therapy is rarely required. The causative agent is *Staphylococcus aureus*.

Conjunctivitis

Primary bacterial conjunctivitis may be gonococcal or chlamydial. Other bacterial infections are relatively uncommon. Gonococcal conjunctivitis may occasionally occur in neonates due to infections from the genital tract at the time of birth. Treatment is by penicillin. The chlamydial infection, trachoma, is an important and serious disease. The causative agent is *Chlamydia trachomatis* serotypes A, B, Ba, and C. It is the commonest cause of blindness in the world and is found where standards of hygiene are low. In some communities the whole population is affected and spread is by flies, hands and contaminated materials. Because of this, although treatment by topical tetracycline is effective, reinfection readily occurs and trachoma remains a widespread illness of worldwide importance. The disease commences as a conjunctivitis, spreads to involve the cornea, and eventually results in corneal scarring.

Milder forms of chlamydial eye infections are seen in developed countries. These are due to *Chlamydia trachomatis* serotypes D–K. Spread is venereal and as in gonococcal conjunctivitis, infection of the infant occurs at the time of birth. The diagnosis is made by staining conjunctival scrapings to show inclusion bodies and the organisms may be cultured by special tissue culture techniques.

Viral conjunctivitis is usually due to adenoviruses and type 8 is particularly associated with outbreaks. Secondary infection with a variety of bacteria may occur and topical chloramphenicol is very useful in the treatment of the bacterial conjunctivitis.

More serious eye infections may occur due to *Herpes zoster* virus. If reactivation of the virus occurs in the trigeminal ganglion and the ophthalmic nerve is affected, there is often eye involvement and this may be sufficiently severe to damage the cornea and seriously affect vision.

Keratitis

Keratitis usually follows direct spread of infection from the conjunctiva. Recurrent *Herpes simplex* infection may take the form of infection of the cornea with the appearance of a dendritic ulcer. Scarring often occurs and the disease tends to be progressive. Treatment is now possible with the antiviral agent idoxuridine.

Endophthalmitis

Endophthalmitis usually occurs only after operations on, or accidental injury to the eye. Treatment is specialized and difficult and involves sub-conjunctival as well as systemic antibiotic administration. A wide variety of organisms may cause endophthalmitis and the choice of antibiotic depends on the sensitivities of the organisms involved.

CHAPTER IV

Infections of the Lower Respiratory Tract

These include bronchitis, bronchiolitis, whooping cough, influenza, pneumonia, tuberculosis, and a variety of less common infections.

BRONCHITIS

Acute Bronchitis

Acute bronchitis is commonly seen in children, often associated with laryngitis and tracheitis. The causative agent is viral, usually para-influenza and influenza viruses. There is often cough with a mucoid sputum and fever. Diagnosis is clinical but the virus may be isolated from the sputum or from a throat swab. Antibiotic therapy is needed only for secondary bacterial infection.

Chronic Bronchitis

This is a common disease occurring in individuals in whom the mucosa has been previously damaged, often by smoking or air pollution. There is an increase in mucus secreting glands in the bronchial mucosa and the disease is characterized by a chronic cough and the production of sputum which initially is mucoid. Exacerbations of the disease occur in the winter months and are associated with the production of purulent sputum. The bacteria associated with the exacerbations are *Haemophilus influenzae* and *Streptococcus pneumoniae*. Treatment is by co-trimoxazole, ampicillin or tetracycline. Antibiotics may usefully be administered for long periods and may be used prophylactically.

The diagnosis is made clinically and laboratory investigations are not very helpful. Isolation of the associated bacteria is useful to determine whether ampicillin resistant *Haemophilus influenzae* strains are present and tuberculosis should be excluded.

71

Bronchiectasis

The symptoms of bronchiectasis are similar to those of chronic bronchitis but this is a more severe disease in which the bronchi are dilated and sac-like. These bronchi are particularly prone to infection and the infecting organisms and the treatment are similar to those of chronic bronchitis.

BRONCHIOLITIS

Bronchiolitis occurs as an acute condition in children up to 2 years of age. Symptoms include wheezing and respiratory obstruction, and the condition may be severe. The causative agent is usually viral, most commonly respiratory syncytial virus. The diagnosis is made clinically but may be confirmed by virus isolation from throat swabs. Treatment is usually symptomatic; antibiotics are not necessary unless there is a secondary bacterial infection.

WHOOPING COUGH

Due to recent anxieties about the complications of whooping cough vaccination, resulting in a smaller number of children being immunized, this disease, which was becoming uncommon, is now regularly seen.

Causative organism

The disease is usually caused by *Bordetella pertussis* and less commonly by *Bordetella parapertussis*. Viral infections may occasionally give rise to a similar clinical picture.

Bordetella pertussis is a small Gram-negative bacillus. Three main serotypes are recognized 1,2: 1,2,3: 1,3. This is important in production of the whooping cough vaccine (Chapter XVIII).

Clinical features

Whooping cough is highly infectious and occurs particularly in younger children. In infants under the age of 6 months it can be an extremely serious and debilitating illness. It is characterized by paroxysms of coughing followed by forced inspiration with the characteristic whoop. The paroxysms of coughing may be followed by vomiting. There may be complications involving the central nervous system. These are haemorrhage due to raised venous pressure, and the results of anoxaemia.

Laboratory Diagnosis

Although the diagnosis of whooping cough is usually made on clinical grounds, it may be confirmed by isolation of the organism. This is best done by sampling the post nasal space using fine per and post nasal swabs. These are plated to an enriched medium, Bordet Gengou, or to charcoal agar. Sometimes a cough plate is used. This is held in front of the mouth during a paroxysm of coughing. As many unwanted organisms are isolated, which may obscure *Bordetella pertussis*, cough plates are now less frequently used.

Prophylaxis

This is by use of a killed vaccine (Chapter XVIII). Because serious complications of vaccination occur, albeit rarely, many parents have been reluctant to have their children vaccinated. However, whooping cough can be a serious infection and modern vaccines are much improved and very safe; vaccination against the disease is therefore recommended.

Treatment

This is generally symptomatic. Tetracycline is useful in the early catarrhal stage of the illness but its usefulness delines after the paroxysms of coughing commence.

INFLUENZA

Influenza is a common illness from which most people suffer on one or more occasions during their lives. This is in part because it is difficult to develop overall immunity to the disease because of antigenic changes undergone by the virus. These are discussed in Chapter XII. Epidemics and indeed pandemics of influenza occur when the immunity of the population is low.

Infecting organisms

These are RNA viruses, the orthomyxoviruses. Influenza A is associated with epidemics of infection; influenza B with sporadic cases.

Clinical features

This is a systemic illness varying considerably in its severity. The symptoms are pyrexia, aching joints and muscles, headache, sore throat and cough. Bronchitis may occur during the course of the illness but the most serious complication is a staphylococcal pneumonia following the viral infection. This may be rapidly fatal but is fortunately rare.

Laboratory diagnosis

No attempt is usually made to make a laboratory diagnosis and because of this, from time to time, more serious illnesses such as brucellosis and subacute bacterial endocarditis are misdiagnosed as influenza.

However, the virus can be isolated from nose and throat swabs and paired sera will show a rise in antibody titre.

Prophylaxis

The difficulties of producing a good vaccine because of the problems of antigenic change have been discussed. Vaccination may be recommended for individuals with chronic respiratory or cardiac disease in whom influenza may be a serious illness. Vaccination is also particularly required in geriatric units where outbreaks may have a high mortality rate. In epidemics, key personnel, doctors, nurses, ambulance men, etc. may be protected.

Treatment

Supportive measures only are required unless secondary bacterial infection supervenes. It is essential that staphylococcal infection is rapidly and effectively treated. Two antibiotics in high dosage are often used. Methicillin and fucidin is a useful combination.

PNEUMONIA

Lobar pneumonia

Typical bacterial lobar pneumonia is becoming increasingly uncommon, probably due to ready antibiotic usage in the early stages of the disease; it is, however, still occasionally seen.

Causative organisms

The typical causative organism of lobar pneumonia is *Streptococcus pneumoniae*, a Gram-positive diplococcus giving characteristic colonies and α haemolysis on blood agar medium. Lobar pneumonia is less commonly due to *Klebsiella pneumoniae*, a capsulate Gram-negative bacillus. Klebsiella pneumonia is less common than pneumococcal pneumonia and occurs particularly in debilitated individuals. Complete resolution following recovery occurs following pneumococcal infection but following klebsiella infection, healing is slow and permanent lung damage results.

Clinical features

The disease is characterized by a rapidly developing inflammatory change usually confined to one lobe. This lobe becomes consolidated and airless, and the patient is breathless and febrile, with a productive cough and rusty sputum. The signs are of consolidation with absent breath sounds and pleurisy is present.

Laboratory diagnosis

This is by the isolation of the causative organism from the sputum.

Prophylaxis

This is of little importance in lobar pneumonia. Pneumococcal vaccines are sometimes used in susceptible individuals, particularly following splenectomy.

Treatment

The treatment of pneumococcal pneumonia is with large doses of benzyl penicillin. Klebsiella pneumonia is more difficult to treat. Combinations of antibiotics may be necessary. Gentamicin is often useful.

Bronchopneumonia

This occurs most commonly at the extremes of age in individuals in whom the lung has been damaged by other diseases such as bronchitis or whooping cough. There is no particular pathogen, a variety of organisms including *Streptococcus pneumoniae* and *Haemophilus influenzae* may be associated with the disease and antibiotic therapy is directed against the predominant organism in the sputum.

Mycoplasma pneumonia

Pneumonia due to *Mycoplasma pneumoniae* does not produce the typical clinical signs of lobar pneumonia seen in pneumococcal infection, but radiological changes may be marked and the illness may last for several weeks. Diagnosis is usually made by demonstrating a rise in antibody level using a complement fixation test although the organism may be isolated. Tetracycline is the treatment of choice.

Psittacosis (ornithosis)

The causative organism is *Chlamydia psittaci* and the disease is usually contracted from psittacine birds (parrots, budgerigars, etc.) but other birds such as turkeys and ducks may be affected (ornithosis). The severity of the disease varies from a mild febrile illness to a severe bronchopneumonia. The diagnosis is made by demonstrating a rising level of antibodies to the organism in a complement fixation test. Treatment is by tetracycline.

Q (Query) Fever

The causative organism is *Coxiella burnetti*. This is a generalized infection and the clinical signs vary but there is often a patchy pneumonia. Man may be infected by drinking contaminated milk or by inhaling dust contaminated with the excreta of infected animals. Again, the diagnosis is made by demonstrating a rising titre of antibodies in a complement fixation test and treatment is by tetracycline.

Legionnaire's disease

This is a disease which has only recently been recognized. The name arose because the disease was first clearly described as an outbreak occurring at a Legionnaires' convention in Philadelphia. The causative agent is *Legionella pneumophila* and the route of infection is by the inhalation of the organism, usually in air contaminated via humidification systems. The organism lives in contaminated water probably in association with a protozoon. The illness, which may be severe, results in a patchy pneumonia. The diagnosis is made by demonstrating a rise in antibody titre using an immunofluorescent test and erythromycin should be given.

Pneumocystis carinii

Pneumocystis pneumonia occurs in debilitated individuals with reduced defences to infection. The exact nature of the organism is unknown. It may be a protozoon or a fungus. It is widely distributed in the human population where it usually gives rise to no symptoms. It is spread by direct personal contact. Diagnosis is usually by biopsy and treatment is by pentamidine.

TUBERCULOSIS

In developed countries there has been during this century a very marked fall in the incidence of tuberculosis. This is predominantly related to improved living standards and better housing, but immunization against the disease and rapid treatment of cases has also helped. In developed countries the disease is more often seen in immigrants from countries where the disease is common, and in people such as vagrants who live in poor conditions. However, it does occur in individuals with no obvious predisposing cause.

Causative organism

This is *Mycobacterium tuberculosis*, a slow growing acid and alcohol fast bacillus which produces characteristic colonies on Loewenstein Jensen medium after 2–6 weeks incubation.

Clinical features

Respiratory tuberculosis in the adult is usually a chronic low grade infection leading to caseation, cavitation, and fibrosis of the lung. The patient may suffer from malaise, weight loss, cough and night sweats. It is important not to overlook the possibility of tuberculosis in elderly patients with chronic bronchitis.

Laboratory diagnosis

The diagnosis of the disease is made in the laboratory by the demonstration of acid and alcohol fast bacilli in the sputum. This is now usually done by staining with lissamine auramine and searching for fluorescing bacilli, but the Ziehl–Neelsen stain may be used.

The presence of acid and alcohol fast bacilli in sputum is almost diagnostic of *M. tuberculosis* infection, but other mycobacteria do occasionally cause lung disease, particularly *M. kansasii*. The sputum, treated to remove other bacteria, is cultured. Loewenstein Jensen medium is commonly used and cultures may become positive in 10 days or may take up to 6–8 weeks. Animal inoculation is not usually required.

Prophylaxis

Prevention of tuberculosis is, as has been indicated, by improvement of living standards, prompt treatment of cases and tracing of contacts and immunization. Before immunization can be carried out, it is necessary to determine whether the individual has already developed immunity to the disease. This is done using the Mantoux test.

If the Mantoux test is negative, immunization may be performed using an attenuated bovine strain of *M. tuberculosis*, Bacille Calmette Guerin (BCG) (Chapter XVIII). In some developed countries BCG vaccination is now reserved for people at high risk of infection.

Treatment

Treatment is specialized and all forms of tuberculosis are best treated by a physician with particular knowledge of the illness. Rifampicin, isoniazid and ethambutol are the antibiotics now commonly used. Once the organism has been isolated, its antibiotic sensitivity should be determined. This is done by incorporating the antibiotics in varying concentrations in Loewenstein Jensen media and looking for the level at which growth no longer occurs. Stringent controls are necessary.

PLEURISY AND PLEURAL EFFUSION

Pleurisy occurs when infection spreads from the lung to involve the pleura. It is regularly seen in pneumococcal pneumonia. There is pain on respiration, and auscultation reveals the characteristic 'pleural rub'. A pleural effusion is a collection of fluid in the pleural cavity. It is seen in a number of conditions including tuberculosis. In that disease examination of fluid removed from the pleural cavity for acid and alcohol fast bacilli may be useful in making a diagnosis.

LUNG ABSCESSES

Lung tissue previously damaged by tuberculosis, chronic bronchitis or bronchiectasis may be invaded by a variety of organisms to give rise to a lung abscess. An aspergilloma occurs when the invading organism is *Aspergillus fumigatus*

PULMONARY ANTHRAX

This is due to inhalation of anthrax spores. It is known as 'wool-sorters' disease (Chapter IX).

CHAPTER V

Infections of the
Central Nervous System

The brain and spinal cord together with their protective membranes and the cerebrospinal fluid (CSF) are normally sterile and are relatively rarely infected. Invasion of them by any micro-organism, bacterial, viral or fungal is liable to result in a serious or even fatal infection.

MENINGITIS

Meningitis is inflammation of the membranes, specifically the pia-arachnoid, covering the brain and spinal cord. It is almost always caused by invasion of the meninges by an infectious micro-organism, although occasionally irritation of the meninges by some other disease process may occur, for example a brain tumour.

The infectious agent gains entry to the sub-arachnoid space via the blood stream and across the blood–CSF barrier or directly from the ear or by way of the nasopharynx, possibly along the sheathes of the olfactory nerves.

The reaction of the meninges may be of two main types, either an acute polymorphic reaction which is the response to attack by most pyogenic bacteria or a lymphocytic reaction to invasion by viruses, spirochaetes, parasites or *Mycobacterium tuberculosis*.

Bacterial Meningitis

Although there is considerable variation from country to country and between different age groups, the most common bacteria to cause meningitis are *Neisseria meningitidis*, *Streptococcus pneumoniae* and *Haemophilus influenzae*. In Britain the meningococcus is the most common cause, followed by the pneumococcus and the haemophilus. More rarely organisms such as coliforms, salmonellae, listeria, staphylo-cocci and β haemolytic streptococci may be involved.

Clinical manifestations

Generally in very young children the onset of the disease is insidious, with no specific signs or symptoms over several days except some pyrexia and a dull unwillingness to feed or to respond. In adults and older children the early stages of the disease are characterized by increasingly severe headache, pyrexia and malaise sometimes with vomiting. In both groups in a few days there is progress to general stiffness of the neck and back with opisthotonos. If untreated the patient may become delirious and lapse into coma. These symptoms may be found in other infections of the CNS such as localized abscesses or even other generalized infections but indicate the need for examination of the CSF by lumbar puncture. This must be done before the commencement of antimicrobial chemotherapy.

Occasionally in adults the onset may be extremely rapid with no preliminary period of malaise. This occurs on occasion in epidemic meningococcal infection. In some meningococcal infections a generalized rash, usually purpuric or petechial in nature, is produced but this is very rare in meningitis due to other organisms.

Laboratory diagnosis

Examination of the Cerebrospinal fluid

This is the only definitive method of diagnosis.

Following lumbar puncture the specimen of CSF should be sufficient (at least 2 ml.) to permit:
  a) observation of its macroscopic appearance;
  b) total red and white cell count;
  c) direct examination of stained smears for micro-organisms;
  d) differential white cell count;
  e) culture of a centrifuged deposit;
  f) estimation of biochemical changes.
The results of these examinations are summarized in Table V.1.

Blood culture

In meningitis blood culture often yields the same organism as that found in the CSF. This is particularly so when the infection is due to meningococci, pneumococci or haemophilus. Blood culture, however, is valuable as another source of diagnosis. In meningococcal infection

Table V.1   Examination of CSF in Meningitis

Nature of Infection	Appearance	White cells ($\times 10^6$/litre)	Protein (g/litre)	Glucose (m.mol/litre)	Common organisms found
Normal	Clear	0–5 lymphocytes	0.2–0.4	2.5–4.7	None
Pyogenic bacterial meningitis	Turbid	1,000–30,000 polymorphs	0.5–5.0	0–2.5	Meningococci, pneumococci, *Haemophilus influenzae*, coliforms, proteus, salmonellae, pseudomonas, klebsiella, staphylococci, streptococci, Listeria
Viral meningitis	Clear	10–1,000 lymphocytes	0.2–5.0	2.5–4.7	Enteroviruses, mumps
Tuberculous meningitis	Clot opalescent	10–1,000 lymphocytes	0.5–5.0	0–2.5	*M. tuberculosis*
Spirochaetal meningitis	Clear	20–2,000 lymphocytes	0.4–5.0	1.0–4.0	*Treponema pallidum, Leptospira icterohaemorrhagiae, Leptospira canicola*

septicaemia may be present without apparent meningeal involvement.

Other diagnostic aids

These include the demonstration of soluble antigen in the CSF by precipitation against antisera in meningococcal infection. Counterimmune electrophoresis and immunofluorescence staining may be used in a variety of infections and may be of some value in rapid diagnosis. Limulus lysate assay may be used to indicate an infection with Gramnegative organisms.

Demonstration of antibodies in the patient's serum is not generally worthwhile in diagnosis of the acute case.

Causative organisms

There are notable variations in the organisms most likely to be involved in meningeal infection, depending on the ages of the patients involved. These are summarized in Table V.2.

Table V.2   Causative Organisms in Meningitis

Age group	Organism
Children	*Haemophilus influenzae, Neisseria meningitidis, Streptococcus pneumoniae*, viruses.
Adults	*Neisseria meningitidis, Streptococcus pneumoniae*, viruses.
Neonates	*Escherichia coli*, other Gram-negative bacilli, streptococcus group B, listeria, staphylococci.
Following trauma (any age)	Staphylococci, streptococci, Gram-negative bacilli, clostridia, bacteroides.

Meningitis in adults and children other than neonates

This group is largely affected by three organisms:
   Neisseria meningitidis
   Haemophilus influenzae
   Streptococcus pneumoniae
Other organisms are comparatively rare.

Meningococcal meningitis

This infection is rarely encountered in patients less than 3 months old and is commonest between 3 months and 5 years, although it also occurs in adults. Mortality is very much higher in patients under 1 year. The infectious process may take a number of widely different forms. Successful invasion of the patient may result in a sudden, overwhelming fulminating septicaemia with shock and circulatory collapse associated with adrenal damage—the Waterhouse–Friederichsen syndrome, there may be meningococcal septicaemia with purpuric rash without circulatory collapse, there may commonly be a presentation of acute meningitis or there may be no evidence of invasion of the bloodstream or the meninges and the colonization may be confined to the naso-pharynx, perhaps causing a rhinitis. Indeed the organism may be carried in the naso-pharynx quite symptomlessly by a small proportion, 1–2%, of healthy individuals.

Meningococcal infections usually occur singly or in small numbers in closely connected groups. This is the 'endemic' situation normally encountered. The disease however may also arise in epidemic form generally in communities living together in considerable numbers as in residential schools, or barrack rooms. Close proximity and poor ventilation may be associated with outbreaks of 'cerebrospinal fever'. In such closed communities the naso-pharyngeal carrier rate of meningococci may be as high as from 20 to 60% without clinical cases of meningitis occurring, but when there is an outbreak the rate of carriage does tend to rise.

Meningococci can be sub-divided serologically into a number of groups. The frequency of occurrence of infection due to these groups varies from country to country but A, B, C, W135 and Y are of most epidemiological importance in the United Kingdom. By far the commonest is group B and the proportion of infections due to it is increasing. Sulphonamide resistance is becoming an increasing problem and is a characteristic of many group A strains and of serotype 2 of group B. This is of importance in prophylaxis, in which sulphonamide is still the drug of choice, although it has largely been superseded in treatment by penicillin.

Laboratory diagnosis

(1) The CSF is generally that of acute pyogenic bacterial meningitis (Table V.1) with classical Gram-negative intracellular diplococci (Fig. V.1) seen on Gram staining. Culture is on chocolate agar with added CO_2.

(2) Blood cultures should be taken and are positive in nearly half of all cases of meningococcal meningitis. The meningococcus may also be

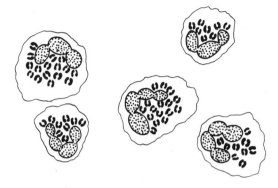

Figure V.1 *Neisseria meningitidis* in CSF. Gram stained

cultured from the naso-pharynx of the patient or from the petechial spots when these are present.

(3) Rapid diagnostic techniques can demonstrate antigens in the CSF by precipitation or counter-immune electrophoresis (Chapter XIX). `

Haemophilus influenzae meningitis

This infection is rare in the neonatal period and occurs almost entirely between 3 months and 3 years, although it does rarely affect older children and adults. The mortality rate is high in untreated cases and is particularly so in babies of under 1 year.

The disease does not occur in epidemics but only in single sporadic cases. The clinical picture is similar to that observed in acute meningococcal meningitis.

Laboratory diagnosis

(1) The CSF will show large numbers of polymorphonuclear leucocytes and varying numbers of small Gram-negative rods, or cocco-bacilli may be seen (Chapter II). These are commonly not intracellular although they may be found within the polymorphs in early stages of the infection. A positive identification of the organism cannot be made on a Gram stained film although, taking the age of the patient into account, an opinion based on probability may be given. Cultures should be made as described above and a growth of small grey translucent colonies may be obtained on blood or chocolate agar. An account of the cultural identification is given in Chapter XIX.

(2) Blood culture is fairly often positive and may be a further aid to diagnosis.
(3) Counter-immune electrophoresis of the CSF can give a rapid indication of the nature of the infection.

Pneumococcal meningitis

This is the second most common form of bacterial meningitis in the United Kingdom. It may occur without apparent precipitating cause or may follow pneumonia or otitis media. It is a particularly serious form of meningitis with a very high mortality. It is most prevalent in children from 3 months to 5 years but is found in older children and in adults. It does not occur in epidemic form but only as sporadic cases.

Laboratory diagnosis

(1) The CSF contains large numbers of polymorphs among which, on Gram staining, the typical Gram-positive lanceolate diplococci may be seen lying extracellularly (Fig. V.2). Special stains may be used to demonstrate the presence of mucoid capsules round the organisms (Chapter II). Culture should be done as described above and within 18 hours should yield the typical α haemolytic 'draughtsman' colonies, although occasionally the growth may be mucoid. Confirmatory tests include optochin testing and bile solubility.

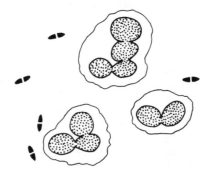

Figure V.2   *Streptococcus pneumoniae* in CSF. Gram stained

(2) Blood culture is positive in a proportion of cases.
(3) Counter-immune electrophoresis may be employed to demonstrate antigens in the CSF.

Neonatal meningitis

An entirely different picture is seen in neonatal meningitis. The patients are of course in the first days, weeks or few months of life. Theirs is much less obviously a meningitic infection and much more a generalized illness, often very difficult to diagnose clinically. They are found to be infected with quite different organisms, most frequently the Gram-negative organisms of the bowel including coliforms, klebsiella, proteus, and pseudomonas. Staphylococci, streptococci, and sometimes *Listeria monocytogenes* are also responsible. This last is a rare cause of meningitis but should be borne in mind particularly where there is immunological deficiency.

Neonates may become infected either during birth, generally with Gram-negative bacteria, or thereafter from their immediate contacts, particularly their attendants. The infection is almost always severe and the mortality is high even with treatment. Neonatal meningitis due to *Streptococcus agalactiae* (Group B streptococcus) is being increasingly recognized as a serious infection in the first month or two of life. The organism, which is also found in the throat, is harboured in the vagina of about a third of normal women and the child is infected usually at birth although it may be infected thereafter. Two separate clinical pictures present themselves. In one, occurring within the first few days of life, there is an acute onset, septicaemia, and a very high mortality. In the other, occurring rather later, meningitis predominates and mortality, although still high, is rather lower. Treatment is with penicillin in high dosage and an aminoglycoside may also be given.

Laboratory diagnosis

(1) The CSF is purulent with large numbers of polymorphs and, on Gram staining, either Gram-negative bacilli, Gram-positive cocci or Gram-positive bacilli may be visible. Culture on the media described will readily yield the appropriate organism although the culture of *Listeria monocytogenes* may be enhanced by first storing the specimen at 4°C for 24–48 hours before culture and by the addition of glucose to the media.
(2) Blood culture is often positive in infection with all these organisms.

Inuries and abnormalities of the CNS

Injury to the skull or spinal column or operative interference ranging from major surgery or implantation of a Spitz Holter drainage valve in hydrocephalus down to simple lumbar puncture may lead to infection of the meninges with a wide variety of organisms. Major congenital abnormalities such as meningomyelocoele also may permit the entry of organisms. These bacteria include not only the common pathogens such as *Staphylococcus aureus*, *Streptococcus pyogenes*, the whole range of enterobacteria, *Clostridium perfringens* and other clostridia, but also less pathogenic 'opportunistic' organisms such as *Staphylococcus albus*, anaerobes such as *Bacteroides* spp. or anaerobic streptococci. The clinical picture ranges from that of acute bacterial meningitis to vague illness when low grade pathogens are involved. Abscesses and other foci may be formed making treatment difficult.

Laboratory diagnosis

(1) The early demonstration and culture of the organism from the CSF concerned is vital so that the appropriate antibiotic treatment may be given. Culture should be aerobic in CO_2 and anaerobic.
(2) If septicaemia co-exists blood culture may be valuable.
(3) Wound swabs from any surface lesion may yield the same organism as that infecting the meninges.
(4) Implants and prostheses such as Spitz-Holter valves may be cultured aerobically in CO_2 and anaerobically.

Tuberculous meningitis

Although this is of course a form of bacterial meningitis it differs markedly from other bacterial infections. Invasion of the meninges by *Mycobacterium tuberculosis* is secondary to some tuberculous infection elsewhere in the body, spread haematogenously or from a local focus, and does not seem to occur in a primary form. It occurs generally in early childhood but may affect adults. The onset is marked by headache and nuchal rigidity but more localized neurological symptoms may predominate, such as convulsion, paralysis or ptosis, depending on the site of the infection and its effect on the circulation of the CSF. The disease progresses to drowsiness, coma, and death unless treated. The organism gives rise not to a polymorphic reaction in the CSF except to some extent in the early stages, but to a lymphocytic one and the sugar level is generally markedly low (table V.1). It is vital that this form of meningitis be distinguished as quickly and urgently as possible from other forms of meningitis characterized by a lymphocytic response, as tuberculous meningitis can and must be treated whereas the other forms due to viruses are generally not fatal and recovery is usually complete without specific treatment.

Laboratory diagnosis

(1) The appearance of the CSF is detailed in Table V.1. Acid alcohol bacilli should be sought and cultivated.
(2) The source of the spread of tuberculosis to the meninges should be sought in the lungs or elsewhere in the body. X-rays and the examination of sputum for *Mycobacterium tuberculosis* should be carried out.

Treatment of bacterial meningitis

Specific diagnosis and proper treatment of bacterial meningitis is dependent on laboratory findings, particularly those in the CSF (Table V.1). An acute pyogenic meningitis, unless in the very early stage, is indicated by large numbers of polymorphs, raised protein and reduced sugar levels. The causative organism may be seen on Gram staining, and the meningococcus and the pneumococcus may be readily identifiable and the appearance of *Haemophilus influenzae* may be sufficiently characteristic to allow an opinion to be given, as may staphylococci and streptococci when they occur. On other occasions, sometimes due to partial treatment or early attempts at diagnosis, it may not be possible to indicate the cause until culture results are available and sometimes not even then. There must be a treatment schedule which can most advantageously be given in meningitis of unknown cause, as well as specific treatment when the cause is known. The age of the patient must also be taken into consideration. It is important for the laboratory to establish the sensitivity of the organism concerned to the chemotherapeutic agents used, especially the sensitivity of the meningococcus to sulphonamides, but in no case must antimicrobial therapy be withheld pending exact diagnosis if meningitis is suspected.

Adults and children other than neonates

1. Initial treatment when the cause is unknown:
   This is still in dispute among clinicians but the most widely accepted choice is:
   (a) Chloramphenicol, which may have rare fatal toxic side effects on the bone marrow; or

(b) Large doses of ampicillin IV.
2. Meningococcal meningitis:
   (a) Benzyl penicillin intramuscularly or intravenously;
   (b) Change to sulphadiazine if the organism is sensitive.
3. Pneumococcal meningitis:
   (a) Benzyl penicillin intravenously at first;
   (b) Thereafter intramuscularly.
4. Haemophilus meningitis:
   (a) Either chloramphenicol intramuscularly or intravenously for 48 hours and thereafter orally; or
   (b) Ampicillin intravenously in high dosage. There is an anomalous effect in that as the inflammation of the meninges improves the drug passes less well into the CSF.

Neonatal meningitis

1. Initial treatment if the cause is unknown should be by gentamicin intramuscularly and intrathecally, and a cephalosporin or benzyl penicillin intravenously or intramuscularly. This regimen should be effective against the most probable cause, the enterobacteriaceae including coliforms, klebsiella and proteus and also pseudomonas, streptococci and staphylococci.
2. If Gram-negative bacilli are seen, gentamicin should be used as above.
3. If Gram-positive cocci are seen, penicillin and cloxacillin should be given. Penicillin and gentamicin may be used for the treatment of infection due to *Streptococcus agalactiae*.
4. Listeria meningitis should be treated with ampicillin intravenously.
5. In all cases sensitivity results from the laboratory must decide the treatment when a specific organism is grown.

Inuries and Abnormalities of the CNS

The treatment which must be instituted depends on any indication given by Gram staining, culture and sensitivity tests.

Tuberculous meningitis

Initially, before sensitivity test results are available, isoniazid should be given together with rifampicin and ethambutol. An alteration in this regimen may be necessary when sensitivity results are known. Treatment should continue for 1 year.

Viral Meningitis

The invasion of the meninges by a virus gives rise to a clinical, pathological, and microbiological picture very different from that produced by bacterial infection.

It is generally caused by an enterovirus (poliovirus, Coxsackie or Echo viruses), mumps virus or the arena virus of lymphocytic chorio-meningitis (LCM). Often meningitis or meningism may accompany or follow viral infections such as measles, german measles and chicken pox but these viruses do not appear in the CSF itself.

Clinical manifestations

There is usually an acute onset of headache and pyrexia, and some degree of rigidity of the neck. There may be sickness and abdominal pain, and conjunctivitis frequently occurs. Normally recovery is spontaneous without specific treatment. Generally the disease is much less severe than bacterial meningitis but of course a very small proportion of those patients infected with poliovirus do progress to damage to the neurones, particularly the anterior horn motor cells of the spinal cord, causing paralysis.

Laboratory diagnosis

Examination of the Cerebrospinal fluid

The fluid is generally clear and the cellular reaction is lymphocytic. The protein is slightly increased and the sugar normal. It is most important at this stage to exclude any possibility of tuberculous meningitis which requires treatment, or other rarer fungal or spirochaetal causes of 'lymphocytic' meningitis.

Culture of the CSF is only rarely successful, apart from infections due to echovirus 9, but the organisms may be isolated from faeces or throat swabs by tissue culture. The cytopathogenic effect of the viruses on tissue culture cells may be seen and the neutralization of this effect by antisera can be used to identify the virus. Coxsackie A viruses can be isolated by the inoculation intracerebrally of suckling mice.

Serology

Confirmation that a certain virus is causing disease must await the demonstration of at least a fourfold rise in antibody titre to that particular virus between an acute stage and a convalescent stage serum.

Treatment

There is no specific treatment for viral meningitis.

ENCEPHALITIS

True encephalitis is viral in origin and often the meninges are also involved to produce meningo-encephalitis. In addition to the picture of meningeal irritation, patients demonstrate confusion, drowsiness and sometimes convulsions.

The groups of viruses involved comprise enteroviruses, which include poliovirus, and coxsackie viruses; the viruses of herpes simplex, rabies, and the wide group of arbo-viruses (arthropod borne) which cause human encephalitis in many parts of the world in addition to many other fevers.

Poliomyelitis

The success of the campaign of immunization against poliomyelitis has much reduced its frequency but it is still seen. The poliovirus has a specific effect on the cells of the anterior horn of the spinal cord, which may result in motor paralysis. In bad cases this can be widespread and permanent.

Herpes

Herpes simplex encephalitis is a serious condition causing necrosis of the brain substance and is often fatal, although treatment can be attempted using cytarabine systemically.

Rabies

Rabies, enzootic in much of the world, invades the CNS via the nerves from the site of an infected animal bite or wound. The importance of prophylactic combined active and passive immunization and of a high level of suspicion in possible cases cannot be too strongly emphasized. Active immunization with inactivated virus grown in human diploid cells should be given if a risk is suspected and protection can be further enhanced by giving passive immunization with specific immune globulin. The wound should be treated at once by thorough washing with soap and the application of iodine. Every effort should be made to identify and if possible to secure the animal involved which should be killed and examined if this is indicated. All animal handlers at special risk should receive prophylactic active immunization before exposure.

Slow Viruses

Two 'slow virus' diseases, kuru and Creutzfeldt–Jakob disease, affect man. They are subacute spongiform encephalopathies and the causative viruses are characterized by very long incubation periods but have not been isolated. Kuru is confined to one New Guinea tribe. It was probably spread by the custom of eating human brain and has nearly disappeared since cannibalism was abandoned among them. Creutzfeldt–Jakob disease is very rare.

OTHER INFECTIONS OF THE CNS

Rare causes of meningitis include cryptococcosis, coccidioidomycosis and histoplasmosis. *Naegleria* spp., an amoeba of soil and water, may cause acute and fatal meningitis in bathers in infected water and the spirochaetes *Leptospira icterohaemorrhagiae* and *Leptospira canicola* can give rise to meningitis as part of the more generalized leptospirosis. *Toxoplasma gondii* may cause meningitis or encephalitis. Syphilis caused by *Treponema pallidum* (Chapter VII) may affect the CNS in a number of ways causing meningitis and other inflammatory changes in the secondary and tertiary stages, and later the development of Tabes dorsalis and General Paralysis of the Insane (GPI). Neurological syphilis causes significant changes in the CSF. The tests normally carried out on serum and described in Chapter VII are positive in syphilitic meningitis. These conditions are much rarer than they used to be due to improved diagnosis and treatment of syphilis in its early stages.

Cryptococcus + candida

BRAIN ABSCESSES

When the substance of the brain is invaded by bacteria a localized abscess is formed rather than generalized encephalitis. The organisms are spread to the brain haematogenously or directly from local sepsis or through trauma. Multiple haematogenously spread abscesses can result from septic emboli from other parts of the body. Otitis media and mastoid infection are common causes of subdural abscess and of sinus thrombosis. Subdural abscesses may be caused by a variety of organisms including staphylococci and aerobic and anaerobic streptococci. They are walled off by gliosis and often defy diagnosis and are very difficult to treat. Sinus thrombosis can give rise to septic emboli.

CHAPTER VI

Urinary Tract Infection

Infections of the urinary tract may involve: the lower tract (bladder and urethra) giving rise to cystitis and urethritis, or the upper tract (kidney) giving rise to glomerulonephritis and pyelonephritis.

LOWER TRACT INFECTION

Cystitis

This is one of the commonest infections seen in domiciliary medical practice. The clinical features include frequency of micturition, dysuria, and supra-pubic discomfort; malaise and pyrexia may occur. It is most often seen in women but it occurs also in men over the age of 50 with obstruction to the bladder outflow due to prostatic hypertrophy. Urinary tract infection (U.T.I.) may, however, occur in all ages and should always be investigated. This is particularly the case with boys because of the regular association in this group of congenital abnormalities with U.T.I.

In hospital patients, U.T.I. follows operative procedures and instrumentation of the urinary tract and its prevention requires high standards of aseptic technique.

Abacterial cystitis (Urethral syndrome)

Women may sometimes suffer from the symptoms of cystitis, but examination of the urine does not reveal a significant bacteriuria. However, it may progress to acute bacterial cystitis. In spite of its name the condition is not due to inflammation of the urethra. It is important to distinguish abacterial from bacterial cystitis as the former does not respond to antibacterial therapy.

Asymptomatic bacteriuria

This is a condition which may occur in females of all ages. Its prevalence is about 5% in adult women, in whom it is generally benign and resolves spontaneously. It is more important in pregnant women, in whom this covert infection may be the first step in a progress to the development of acute pyelonephritis. For this reason routine screening of pregnant women for bacteriuria should be carried out so that early treatment can be given. In children kidney damage may also occur following infection, mainly in those below 5 years of age. This is particularly likely to happen if urine ascends the ureters when the bladder contracts. This is known as vesico-ureteric reflux. The early detection and treatment of urinary tract infection in young children is valuable in the prevention of renal damage.

In patients with abnormalities of the renal tract, the long term consequences of infection may also be severe.

Laboratory diagnosis

The essential criterion for the laboratory diagnosis of U.T.I. is the presence in freshly voided urine of 10^5 or more organisms/ml. Contaminating organisms originally present in small numbers (10^3 or less) will multiply in the urine after it has been passed. For this reason the types of specimen examined and the method of transport to the laboratory are important.

Types of specimen

Mid-stream urine (M.S.U.)

This is the commonest type of specimen examined. To obtain good specimens of this type may be difficult in women but provided that obvious contamination is avoided, reasonably satisfactory urine samples may be obtained.

Catheter specimen urine

Catheterization itself predisposes to the development of U.T.I., so catheter specimens are used only when the patient is already catheterized for some other reason.

'Bag' specimens of urine

It may be difficult to obtain good specimens of urine from infants. With luck a specimen may be 'caught'. If not, a specimen passed into a bag attached to the perineum may be used and is satisfactory if the bag is emptied frequently.

Supra-public aspiration of urine

If it is difficult to obtain a suitable M.S.U., urine may be collected directly from the bladder by aspiration. This is most commonly done in infants in whom the bladder is an abdominal organ.

Ureteric specimens

These may be obtained during the course of an operation. They are valuable specimens because they can be used to distinguish between upper and lower tract infection and to determine whether both kidneys are involved.

Early-morning specimens of urine

These are used for the diagnosis of renal tuberculosis. At least three specimens should be examined.

Terminal specimens of urine

The terminal part of the urine specimen is sometimes recommended for examination for the presence of the parasite *Schistosoma haematobium*.

Transport to the laboratory

This is arranged so that multiplication of bacteria in the urine does not occur.

Rapid transport

This is generally impracticable.

Refrigeration

The urine may be collected in a clean sterile container and refrigerated until examined.

Borate bottles

The urine may be collected in a bottle containing borate. This will, for most bacterial species, maintain the bacterial count at the same level for 24 hours or more.

Dip-slide

A slide coated in nutrient media is dipped into the urine as soon as it is passed, drained and then placed in a sterile container and sent to the laboratory where it can be incubated.

Examination in the laboratory

White blood cells

In the absence of information about the patient's fluid intake and the time over which the specimen has been collected, assessment of the significance of numbers of white cells in the urine becomes difficult. Centrifugation of the urine with re-suspension of the deposit in a small volume of urine may be used but does introduce even more variables. The presence in uncentrifugated urine of more than 10 white cells per high power field of the microscope may be taken as indicating an abnormally high number of white cells, which is often due to the presence of infection.

Red blood cells

The same preparation may be used to demonstrate the presence of red blood cells. These may be present in small numbers in the presence of infection, particularly infection with *M. tuberculosis*. Large numbers of red cells may be due to bleeding into the urinary tract or to acute nephritis.

Culture of urine

The aim of urine culture is to determine whether bacteria are present, and if so, the number and whether they are in pure culture. This is usually achieved by semi-quantitative culture on MacConkey or CLED medium. Semi-quantitative culture may be done by using a loop which delivers a known volume of urine. For rapid screening of large numbers of urines, many of which will be sterile, a strip of filter paper may be used to inoculate the media (Fig. VI.1).

Dip slides have already been described. They are particularly useful if specimens have to be transported long distances to the laboratory.

The results are usually reported as:

significant:	10^5 or more organisms/ml;
of doubtful significance:	10^4 organisms/ml;
not significant:	10^3 or less organisms/ml.

The organisms reported as 'not significant' are contaminants which enter the urine at the time of collection and may subsequently multiply. If the urine is properly collected and stored, 10^5 organisms/ml or more indicate infection.

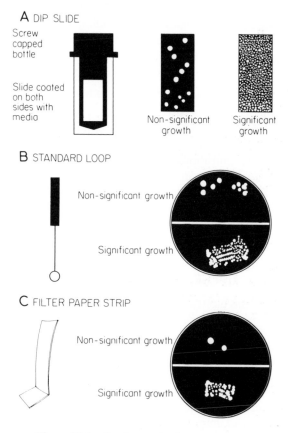

Figure VI.1 Semi-quantitative urine culture

Organisms which cause urinary tract infection

Urinary tract infections are generally ascending, the source of the organism being the patient's own bowel. *Escherichia coli* is the commonest cause of urinary tract infection, particularly in patients outside hospital. Other organisms regularly isolated from urine include enterococci, proteus, pseudomonas, micrococci (Group 3), and klebsiella spp. Organisms showing multiple resistance to antibiotics, particularly pseudomonas and klebsiellas are more commonly found in hospital in-patients, particularly following surgery or instrumentation.

In many laboratories identification of urinary pathogens is based primarily on colonial appearance. This is generally adequate for clinical purposes, detailed biochemical identification not usually yielding useful information other than for epidemiological investigations. However, it must be remembered that salmonellas, including *Salmonella typhi*, may be present in the urine, and colonies of non-lactose fermenting organisms that are not proteus should be identified.

Antibiotic sensitivity determinations

As well as the commonly used antibiotics such as ampicillin and trimethoprim-sulphonamide, urinary antiseptics, nalidixic acid, and nitro-furantoin are also available. Antibiotics may be concentrated in the urine so higher concentrations of antibiotics than usual are used in the antibiotic discs used for sensitivity testing.

Some bacteria may be resistant to the commonly used antibiotics, particularly if the patient has been hospitalized or has undergone surgery, and it may sometimes be necessary to carry out sensitivity testing to gentamicin and other amino-glycosides.

UPPER TRACT INFECTIONS

These include glomerulonephritis and acute and chronic pyelonephritis.

Glomerulonephritis

The commonest form of glomerulonephritis occurs 10–20 days following acute streptococcal infection, which may be of the throat or skin. Unlike rheumatic fever, a limited number of types of streptococci are responsible and therefore recurrences are rare. The disease is not due to the infection itself but rather to an immunological response to infection. A number of mechanisms have been implicated; these include circulating soluble toxic complexes which are filtered off in the glomerulus and the production of anti-glomerular basement membrane antibody. The patient suffers from oedema due to fluid retention, haematuria, and there may be loin pain and malaise. Rarely, the disease may be so severe as to lead to renal failure.

Laboratory investigations

Examination of the urine will show the presence of red blood cells. There may be no other abnormality.

Serological investigations will show the presence of a raised ASO (anti streptolysin 'O') titre. There is a raised level of antibodies to the oxygen-labile haemolysin produced by streptococci. A high titre indicates only that there has been recent streptococcal infection.

Acute pyelonephritis

This is almost always an ascending infection from the bladder and is most likely to occur when there is obstruction to outflow. The organisms associated with acute pyelonephritis are the same as those causing cystitis. The symptoms also are similar, but systemic manifestations are more common and more severe, and loin pain may be present.

Laboratory investigations

The laboratory diagnosis of acute pyelonephritis is similar to that of acute cystitis. Distinguishing between upper and lower tract infection in the laboratory may be attempted. The examination of ureteric specimens if these are available is useful. Similar information may be obtained by examination of catheter specimens of urine following bladder washout and during a diuresis (Fairley technique). Under these circumstances the bladder urine is similar to a ureteric specimen. It may sometimes be useful to determine the titre of serum antibodies to the infecting organism. Generally this is higher in upper than in lower tract infection. However, the results are often not clear cut and are only useful in confirming the site of infection when taken in conjunction with the clinical signs and the radiological evidence.

Chronic pyelonephritis

Acute pyelonephritis may sometimes proceed to chronic disease but the relationship between the two conditions is obscure and chronic pyelonephritis is often found without a history of preceding acute disease. The factors predisposing to chronic pyelonephritis include: the presence of renal scars before the age of 4 years, vesico-ureteric reflux, and persistent or recurrent infection.

Laboratory investigations

The laboratory findings are often not helpful in making a diagnosis as there may not be significant bacteriuria and white cell excretion may be little changed.

Renal failure

Any degree of impairment of renal function is important in administration of antibiotics excreted by the kidney. Gentamicin gives rise to most problems, in part because it is itself nephrotoxic, but also because the gap between the therapeutic and toxic levels is narrow with this antibiotic.

In patients on haemodialysis, the bacteriological problems consist of prevention of infection at the catheter site and correct maintenance of the dialysis equipment. In chronic ambulatory peritoneal dialysis, prevention of peritonitis is extremely important because loss of the dialysing surface occurs following infection. This is probably best done by extremely careful aseptic technique and detailed instruction of patients.

Tuberculosis of the renal tract

Renal tuberculosis is said to present in the laboratory as a 'sterile pyuria', that is a urine which contains pus cells but from which bacterial pathogens are not isolated by conventional culture techniques. Haematuria is usually also present and in practice, secondary bacterial infection often also occurs. If tuberculosis is suspected on clinical or laboratory grounds, the urine deposit is stained for tubercle bacilli and cultures are set up. It should be remembered that although the presence of acid and alcohol fast bacilli in sputum is almost diagnostic of tuberculosis, the possibilities of contamination of urine with non-pathogenic mycobacteria are greater, although even in urine this does not frequently occur.

Schistosomiasis

This is a geographically widespread infection affecting many people in Asia, Africa, and South America. *Schistosoma haematobium* infection is the form of the disease in which the bladder is involved. The life cycle of the parasite is shown in Fig. VI,2. The adults live in the vesical venous

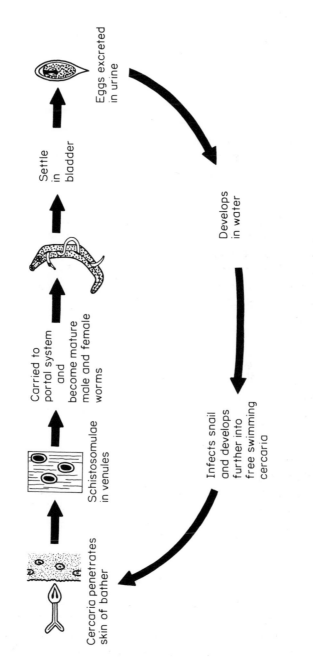

Figure VI.2 Life cycle of *Schistosoma haemotobium*

plexus and the ova are extruded into the bladder. Characteristically the urine contains blood and the schistosoma ova; again secondary infection may be present.

Candidiasis

This may occur as part of a systemic infection or as an ascending infection from a bladder catheter. In the latter case, removal of the catheter is required. In systemic infections 5-fluorocytosine or amphotericin may be used (Chapter VI).

CHAPTER VII

Venereal Diseases and Infections of the Genital Tract

This chapter considers the venereal diseases together with non-venereal infections of the body caused by closely related organisms. It also includes genital tract infections in general whether venereal or not.

SYPHILIS

Venereal Syphilis

Clinical disease

This generalized systemic infection is caused by the *Treponema pallidum*, a spirochaete, passed almost always directly from person to person during sexual intercourse. The infection is regarded as having several phases.

(1) Primary

After a symptomless incubation period of about 3 weeks during which the spirochaete spreads in the bloodstream throughout the body, a 'chancre' appears on the genital area. This primary sore forms a painless ulcerating nodule, accompanied by swelling of the inguinal glands. It may alternatively be found in the mouth or rectum following contact with these parts in oral or anal receptive sex. It persists for some weeks before healing.

(2) Secondary

The primary stage is further followed within 1 or 2 months by the appearance of secondary lesions in the form of a skin rash, usually macular or papular, and the development of shiny white thickened patches on the mucosa of the mouth. The skin rash is characteristically symmetrical in distribution and it often affects the palms of the hands and the soles of the feet. Papules in the vulval and perineal area are known as condylomata lata. The patient may feel generally unwell and have a low grade pyrexia. This stage of the disease does not last more than a few months after which the symptoms subside.

(3) Tertiary

This stage only manifests itself in about a third of untreated affected patients and appears a variable number of years after the initial infection. It affects the cardiovascular system and the central nervous system, or may develop as a chronic granulomatous process or gumma affecting any organ of the body, often bone, testis or liver. Cardiovascular syphilis is due to the effect of the treponema on the arterioles in the adventitia and the media of vessel walls. This leads to fibrosis and even necrosis of the media. The aorta is most often affected and the process may go on to the formation of an aneurysm. In the central nervous system, at this stage, syphilis affects the meninges, sometimes leading to gumma formation.

(4) Quaternary

Neurosyphilis with clinical manifestations can occur in a few untreated cases as long as 10, 20 or 30 years after infection. In meningovascular syphilis the lesion is inflammatory causing endarteritis obliterans of the small arteries of the cortex with thrombosis and ischaemia. Parenchymatous neurosyphilis involves a destruction of the nerve cells themselves and may be widespread with encephalitis in General Paralysis of the Insane. This involves paresis together with changes of intellect and personality. The eye is affected to give the small irregular Argyll–Robertson pupil which reacts to accommodation but not to light. The spinal cord is the site of damage in Tabes dorsalis with degeneration of the posterior roots both inside and outside the cord. The main symptoms are locomotor ataxia and disturbed sensory function with paraesthesia and sometimes acute shooting or 'lightning' pains. The tendon reflexes can be absent and there is bladder disturbance and sexual impotence.

These late manifestations of syphilis, although occurring only in a small percentage of untreated cases, were once quite commonly seen. They are rare today because of the success of treatment of syphilis in its earlier stages.

Laboratory diagnosis

Direct microscopy

The spirochaete *Treponema pallidum* may be demonstrated in the exudate from the primary chancre, in aspirations from local lymph nodes, from the lesions in the mucosa or from condylomata lata. The treponema is seen either by dark-ground or phase contrast microscopy as an actively motile fine spirochaete about 10 μ in length and 0.2 μ in breadth, with about 10 primary spirals. It moves actively to and fro showing rotation and flexion. It is best seen in fresh exudate in the ward or clinic but diagnosis cannot be assured by this method alone as other spirochaetes may be present and can be difficult to distinguish from *Treponema pallidum*. Specific fluorescent antibody staining can be used to aid diagnosis.

Serology

Lipoidal antigen tests

The diagnosis of syphilis by demonstrating the presence of antibodies in the patient's serum can easily be divided into those tests which demonstrate a non-specific antibody or reagin which reacts with an alcohol soluble lipoidal antigen and those demonstrating a specific treponemal antibody. Many of the tests based on lipoidal antigen are of historic interest only, including the Wasserman reaction or WR, a complement fixation test, and the Kahn test, a flocculation test. The non-specific cardiolipin test now used is the VDRL or Venereal Disease Research Laboratory test. This is a valuable screening test which becomes positive during the primary stage of syphilis, usually about a week after infection. As it is non-specific, positive reactions can be given in other conditions. These include normal pregnancy, infections both bacterial and viral, malaria and connective tissue diseases such as Systemic Lupus Erythematosus. Such reactions are known as 'Biological False Positives'.

The VDRL test employs a cardiolipin antigen prepared as an alcoholic extract of heart muscle together with lecithin and cholesterol. This is mixed on a slide with the patient's serum and flocculation is observed in positive tests. The test can be done as a quantitative test by using doubling dilutions of the patient's serum to provide an end point after which there is no flocculation.

Treponemal antigen tests

The Reiter Protein Complement Fixation Test (RPCFT) was at one time useful in diagnosis using an antigen prepared from ultrasonicated non-pathogenic Reiter treponemes. It therefore avoided the biological false positives shown in lipoidal antigen tests but it could not be regarded as specific for infection with *Treponema pallidum* as it reacted with any treponemal antibody.

The Fluorescent Treponemal Antibody-Absorbed Test (FTA-ABS) uses an antigen obtained from the *Treponema pallidum* itself but it still gives cross-reactions with other treponemes. These, however, are screened out as far as possible by absorption of anti-treponemal group antibodies from the patient's serum by a Reiter treponeme preparation so that the test is quite specific. It becomes positive early in primary syphilis and remains positive in secondary, tertiary and quaternary syphilis. It is quantitative in that the degree of fluorescence in the test is compared with control sera of known reaction from weak to very strong positive. This is an indirect test for the presence of specific immunoglobulin. In positive tests after the initial reaction in which the serum antibodies are bound to the treponemes, their presence is demonstrated by combination with an anti-human immunoglobulin conjugated with fluorescein (Chapter XIX).

The *Treponema pallidum* Haemagglutination Test (TPHA) also uses an antigen obtained from *Treponema pallidum* itself. This is used to sensitize formalinized, tanned sheep red cells, and the agglutination of these coated cells is compared against that of uncoated cells when mixed with the serum of the patient in microtitre plate wells.

The *Treponema pallidum* Immobilization Test (TPI)—for many years the undisputed definitive test for treponemal infection, this test is technically very complicated, requiring the maintenance of live spirochaetes. It is less sensitive than the FTA-ABS test and is not often positive in primary syphilis. It is now confined to a few laboratories and is little used. It does not distinguish between infections due to *Treponema pallidum* and those due to other treponemes.

Interpretation of laboratory tests

The standard tests used now are the VDRL, the FTA-ABS and the TPHA.

Primary syphilis

Reagin tests will be positive. The FTA-ABS and TPHA will become positive during the primary stage. Successful treatment at this stage will result in all tests becoming negative.

Secondary syphilis

All tests will be positive. Treatment will result in reagin tests becoming negative but the treponemal tests remain positive.

Tertiary syphilis

All tests are usually positive, although reagin tests sometimes become negative. Treatment will result in any positive reagin tests becoming negative but treponemal tests remain positive.

Biological false positives may occur with reagin tests and they therefore can never be definitive. Their great value is as a simple screening test with confirmation by a treponemal antigen test, and in the early primary stage of syphilis when with clinical evidence or the presence in a chancre of spirochaetes morphologically resembling *Treponema pallidum* they can give confirmation of a diagnostic suspicion.

All tests can be positive in Yaws or Pinta.

Treatment

The treatment of syphilis at any stage is based on establishing adequate penicillin levels over a period of 10 days by giving 600,000 units daily of procaine penicillin intramuscularly. In late syphilis it is advisable to continue treatment for 2 weeks. In penicillin allergy, tetracycline, erythromycin or cephalosporins may be used. Treatment can be complicated by a pyrexial reaction to the damaged treponemes, the Jarisch–Herxheimer reaction.

Congenital Syphilis

A syphilitic mother will transmit the infection across the placenta to her unborn child. The foetus may be stillborn particularly if the maternal infection is recent.

Subsequent live births may be infected and show lesions of congenital syphilis in infancy. These include rhinitis, skin rashes and sloughing particularly on the palms and the soles of the feet and around the mouth, nose and anus. The bones are affected, noticeably the nasal bone and the legs, giving 'saddle nose' and 'sabre shins', while the incisor teeth are peg shaped. Other organs such as the lungs, liver and kidneys are also involved in this generalized infection.

Treatment is by procaine penicillin, 50,000 units/kg daily intramuscularly for 10 days. Untreated cases can progress to neurosyphilis, joint arthropathy and corneal keratitis leading to blindness.

Endemic Syphilis

This non-venereal form of syphilis is caused by the *Treponema pallidum* and affects hot dry areas of the Sahara, Sudan, East Africa, the Middle East, Central Asia, and Central Australia. It is a contagious disease easily passed particularly among children in poor crowded conditions.

It is rarely seen in the primary stage and usually first appears as a secondary macular or papular rash affecting especially the mouth and pharynx and the moist flexures, perineal, perianal and axillary areas of the body. There may be periostitis and lymphadenopathy.

The disease usually enters a latent period but a further tertiary stage with gummata, hyperkeratosis, periostitis, and de-pigmentation of the skin may follow. The disease does not usually affect the central nervous system or the cardiovascular system. Serological diagnosis and treatment are closely similar to venereal syphilis.

YAWS

This disease is caused by *Treponema pertenue*, a spirochaete indistinguishable morphologically or serologically from *Treponema pallidum*. Yaws, however, occurs only in the tropics and is a contagious nonvenereal infection. The primary stage after the treponeme has entered through some break in the skin is a raised granular papilloma or an ulcer. A latent phase then precedes the secondary stage with papular skin rash affecting all parts of the body and often appearing in papillomatous forms resembling a raspberry, giving rise to the name Framboesia for the disease. Osteitis and periostitis are also seen. In the tertiary stage gummata and hyperkeratosis occur.

Serological diagnosis is as for syphilis. Treatment is by penicillin, usually as a single dose of 1.2 mega unit procaine penicillin in oil. The disease may disappear spontaneously.

PINTA

This disease occurs in South and Central America and is due to *Treponema carateum* which is morphologically and serologically indistinguishable from *Treponema pallidum*. It is contagious, passing from person to person by contact of the exudate from a skin lesion with broken skin. The papular lesions are itchy and tend to spread. In the secondary stage there are more spreading papular rashes (Pintids) with lymphadenitis and in the tertiary stage changes in pigmentation occur. The disease does not affect the body generally and there are no changes in the central nervous system or cardiovascular system.

Serological diagnosis is as for syphilis and treatment is by penicillin as for Yaws.

GONORRHOEA

Infecting organism

This disease is due to infection with *Neisseria gonorrhoeae*. This Gram-negative, oxidase positive diplococcus is a member of the same family as *Neisseria meningitidis*. It can be differentiated by its fermentation of sugars from other neisseria.

Clinical condition

The organism is usually spread by sexual intercourse or other sexual intimacy. In the male 2–9 days after exposure it gives rise to dysuria and inflammation of the mucosa of the urethra with a purulent discharge in which the organisms can be found often within polymorphonuclear leucocytes—the typical intracellular Gram-negative diplococcus. The disease is usually self limiting even without treatment but it may rarely involve the epididymis of the testis, or the prostate and seminal vesicles, and become a chronic infection or carrier state.

In the female the disease presents as a urethritis or cervicitis and rarely as a vaginitis. Symptoms often are minimal and there may be no complaint or even awareness of the disease. This increases the danger of further spread to other sexual partners. In a small percentage of cases the disease may spread to involve Bartholin's glands and even the endometrium and the fallopian tubes. This salpingitis may be a cause of later infertility.

Very occasionally the infection in either sex may become systemic. The organism has a predilection for joints and tendon sheaths and can cause arthritis and synovitis.

Other sites of infection include the rectum, particularly in male homosexuals, the mouth and pharynx in both sexes and the eye in neonates infected from their mother's genital tract or in adults by poor hygiene and direct transfer by hand to eye. Neonatal conjunctivitis or ophthalmia due to the gonococcus must be treated at once by intensive use of penicillin.

Female infants and little girls may suffer from vulvo-vaginitis following sexual contact or assault. This condition may also spread among young girls in wards and institutions due to communal sharing of towels and bad hygiene.

Treatment

The gonococcus normally is extremely sensitive to penicillin and most other common antibiotics. It is now sadly often resistant to sulphonamides. The treatment of choice is benzyl penicillin, 5 mega units IM, or procaine penicillin, 4.8 mega units IM, preceded in both cases by 1g probenecid orally to increase peak levels by delaying excretion. A single dose of these agents is generally sufficient. Kanamycin 2g or spectinomycin 2g given once intramuscularly can be used in cases of penicillin allergy or penicilling resistance. The proportion of gonococci resistant to penicillin varies from place to place but is increasing. β-lactamase producing organisms which first originated in the Far East and West Africa are now widely distributed and concurrent spectinomycin resistance has been reported.

It is important that gonococci are cultured and their sensitivity tested. Oral agents such as tetracycline and cotrimoxazole can be used with the disadvantage of dependence on the patient not to default on treatment.

Neonatal ophthalmia is treated by penicillin in high doses intravenously for at least 1 week.

CHLAMYDIA TRACHOMATIS INFECTIONS

The infecting organism

The chlamydiae are a form of bacteria which are unusual in being obligate intracellular parasites unable to synthesize high energy compounds.

Clinical conditions

Certain serotypes A, B, Ba and C of *Chlamydia trachomatis* are the cause of trachoma, an eye infection (Chapter III).

Serotypes D-K are the cause of urethritis which is venereally transmitted and serotype L gives rise to lymphogranuloma venereum.

Chlamydial urethritis

It is difficult to evaluate the significance of the presence of *Chlamydia trachomatis* in the urethra. It is found in the urethra in some men who are symptom free but it is also more frequently found in non-gonococcal urethritis (NGU) and its presence in these cases may be associated with a rise in the titre of serum antibodies to it. It is also frequently isolated from the cervix of asymptomatic women but again is more frequently found in cervicitis and may also cause urethritis and salpingitis. In men epididymitis is a complication.

Chlamydia trachomatis is frequently found together with *Neisseria gonorrhoeae* in urethritis. Treatment of the condition with penicillin will leave the chlamydia unaffected and give rise to 'post-gonococcal urethritis'.

Diagnosis is by tissue culture of scrapings or exudate, when the inclusion bodies can be seen. Demonstration of a rising titre in the patient's serum by fluorescence or the presence of IgM antibodies are diagnostic tests in urethritis and salpingitis.

Lymphogranuloma venereum

This disease is spread by sexual contact. The first manifestation is a small, quickly healing, ulcer on the penis or in women on the external genitalia or vagina. Two weeks later there is progressive enlargement of the inguinal or pelvic lymph nodes followed by breakdown and discharge. The condition may continue for many weeks, and complications include rectal stricture due to scarring.

Treatment

Tetracyclines have been most widely used in treatment, being given for 2 to 3 weeks. Other agents such as sulphonamides, erythromycin or chloramphenicol have also been advocated.

GRANULOMA INGUINALE

Infecting organism

This is a small pleomorphic Gram-negative rod, often encapsulated, which does not grow on laboratory media on first isolation and should be cultivated in the yolk sac of chick embryos. Long known as *Donovania granulomatis* it is now defined as *Calymmatobacterium granulomatis*. It may be seen in exudate from an ulcer as typical capsulated bipolar staining 'Donovan bodies' inside large macrophages.

Clinical condition

The infection is generally spread venereally and is more common in the tropics, producing ulcerating papules of the genitalia after an incubation period usually of about a week. The lesions spread outwards involving the genitalia, the perineum, the thighs and the rectum. There is extensive scar tissue with strictures and the formation of fistulas. Lymph drainage may be blocked and secondary infection is very common.

Treatment

A course of tetracycline or ampicillin over 2 or more weeks or of streptomycin over 1 week is usually successful.

CHANCROID

Infecting organism

Haemophilus ducreyi, a Gram-negative bacillus, can be demonstrated in smears from the lesions and isolated in culture.

Clinical condition

This venereal disease results within a few days of exposure in the formation of a papule, typically tender, on the genitalia. This develops to a painful ulcer, often with local lymphadenitis.

Treatment

Sulphonamides or tetracycline are the drugs of choice, although streptomycin can be used.

GENITAL MYCOPLASMOSIS

Infecting organism

Two organisms of the Mycoplasmataceae family are found involved in infections of the genital tract, *Mycoplasma hominis* and *Ureaplasma urealyticum*.

Clinical conditions

The true role of these organisms in genital infections is as yet not established. *Ureaplasma urealyticum* is found associated with non-gonococcal urethritis and *Mycoplasma hominis* has been demonstrated in vaginitis and other genital inflammations. There seems little doubt that they can be passed venereally.

Treatment

Both agents are sensitive to tetracycline. *Ureaplasma urealyticum* is also sensitive to erythromycin and *Mycoplasma hominis* to lincomycin.

VAGINITIS

Inflammatory conditions with vaginal discharge occur commonly due to simple infectious agents. These may form part of the normal flora of the body and act as opportunistic pathogens during an alteration of conditions due perhaps to hormonal changes or antibiotic therapy, or may be introduced during intercourse. Gonorrhoea has been discussed previously.

Trichomonal Vaginitis

Infecting organisms

The *Trichomonas vaginalis* is a pear-shaped motile flagellated parasite measuring about $25 \times 15 \mu$. It has a single nucleus at the anterior end and four anterior flagella with a fifth at the tip of a lateral undulating membrane (see Fig. I,6). It is found in the vagina and also in the male urethra.

Clinical conditions

The infection is transmitted venereally. Acute vaginitis may occur with copious frothy discharge or the infection may be more chronic. The parasite can be recognized in wet preparations made from vaginal swabs or may be cultured in special liquid media.

Treatment

The most effective treatment is with metronidazole 200 mg three times a day for a week.

Vaginal Candidiasis (Moniliasis)

Infecting organism

Candida albicans is a yeast normally seen as a large oval Gram-positive cell about 3 μ in diameter. It is commonly found in many sites of the body including the mouth, vagina, intestine, and skin.

Clinical conditions

Clinical infection may follow some alteration in the normal conditions of the environment of the organism. It is an outstandingly successful opportunistic pathogen, especially following prolonged broad spectrum antibiotic thereapy, when it thrives in the absence of competitive organisms, causing intestinal moniliasis or thrush of the mouth.

Monilial vaginitis is characterized by a thick white discharge, itching, and the formation of white patches on the mucous membrane. The organism can be readily seen in direct microscopy and is easily cultured from swabs of the discharge. Its presence is not diagnostic as it is a common normal inhabitant.

Treatment

Local treatment using nystatin pessaries is best and may be continued for 10–15 days.

Vaginitis due to other Causes

Many organisms may be found in the vagina both in health and in the presence of vaginitis. These include the staphylococci and the common organisms of the bowel such as coliforms, *Streptococcus faecalis* and anaerobic organisms. The significance of these is difficult to assess.

Corynebacterium vaginale

An organism recently more specifically associated with vaginitis and vaginal discharge is *Corynebacterium vaginale (Haemophilus vaginalis)*. This is probably sexually transmitted and gives rise to a relatively mild vaginitis. It may be suggested by the presence of 'Clue cells' with small Gram-negative cocco-bacilli adhering to the surface of vaginal epithelial cells. The condition responds to treatment with metronidazole.

Streptococcus agalactiae

This group B streptococcus is aerobic, weakly β-haemolytic and is being increasingly reported as a cause of serious neonatal infection including meningitis and pneumonia. It is found in the genital tract of a significant proportion of women, from where it colonizes the newborn infant. It may be found in association with vaginitis and it may be passed venereally. It is sensitive to penicillin and most common antibiotics.

Herpes genitalis

This viral infection of the genitalia is predominantly due to *Herpes simplex* type 2, while type 1 is generally associated with oral lesions. Multiple vesicles appear on the external genitalia and may be extremely tender. They eventually crust over and heal but may go on to cervicitis. Diagnosis is by inoculation of vesicle fluid into tissue cultures and the demonstration of a cytopathic effect. Serum antibody may be demonstrated by complement fixation but it is difficult to evaluate as most adults have been infected. Antiviral drugs such as idoxuridine have an effect on *Herpes simplex* virus and may be used in serious cases or in pregnancy.

SALPINGITIS

The fallopian tubes are most often infected by spread of organisms from the vagina via the endometrium, although spread from the peritoneum may also occur and the tubes may also be infected in generalized infections such as tuberculosis.

Inflammation with production of a purulent exudate commonly occurs in gonococcal infection. Acute salpingitis may progress to a chronic stage and result in sterility. This outcome is almost inevitable in tuberculous infection. Early treatment with appropriate agents is important.

ORCHITIS, EPIDIDYMITIS, AND PROSTATITIS

Infection of the testis and the epididymis can follow infection of the urethra or the bladder with either gonococci or the organisms of urinary infection such as coliform bacilli. The infection can cause destruction of the testicular tissue with consequent sterility.

Chlamydia trachomatis has been found in significant numbers of cases of epididymitis.

Tuberculous epididymitis is a frequent complication of tuberculosis of the renal tract. It may lead to complete destruction of the epididymis.

Orchitis is a rare complication of brucellosis.

Epididymo-orchitis is a common complication of mumps in men above the age of puberty. It is generally unilateral and gives rise to enlargement and tenderness. It rarely can lead to sterility in bilateral infections.

The prostate is also involved in spread of infection from the urethra. Gonococci give rise to acute prostatitis, generally becoming chronic. The organisms of urinary tract infection may also spread to give acute or suppurative prostatitis.

CHAPTER VIII

Infections of the
Gastro-intestinal Tract

In this chapter we include infections of the mouth as well as food poisoning, dysentery, gastro-enteritis in infants, travellers' diarrhoea, enteric fever, cholera, and pseudo-membranous colitis.

INFECTIONS OF THE MOUTH

Oral candidiasis

The causative agent of this condition is *Candida albicans*. It occurs in infants and the debilitated, and following antibiotic administration. It is characterized by the formation of white plaques on the mucous membrane. Treatment is by nystatin lozenges.

Vincent's angina

This is a painful ulcerative condition of the mouth and throat; it is diagnosed by finding large numbers of spirochaetes *Borrelia vincentii* together with fusiform bacteria in the Gram-stained smear of the lesion. The fusiform bacteria are anaerobic and metronidazole is effective in treatment as also is penicillin.

FOOD POISONING

The term 'food poisoning' is loosely used to describe those conditions in which bacteria or their products are ingested in food and cause disease which is usually limited to the gastro-intestinal tract. It is not used to describe systemic diseases such as the enteric fevers or predominantly water-borne diseases like cholera. The types of food poisoning to be considered are those caused by salmonellas, campylobacters, *Staphylococcus aureus*, *Clostridium perfringens*, *Bacillus cereus*, *Vibrio parahaemolyticus*, and *Clostridium botulinum*. All except *Clostridium botulinum* cause symptoms directly related to the gastro-intestinal tract, such as vomiting, diarrhoea, and abdominal pain. There are differences in the relative importance of these and in the time of onset following ingestion of the contaminated food.

Salmonella food poisoning

A large number of strains of salmonellas may cause food poisoning. It is predominantly a disease of animals spread to the human population via contaminated food. The organism enters the kitchen on raw meat and poultry and is either not destroyed due to inadequate cooking, or cross-contamination of cooked food from raw occurs. Whatever the source of contamination, outbreaks of infection are more likely to occur if the food is left at a temperature at which the organisms will multiply. The methods of prevention of salmonella food poisoning are obvious: food must be cooked sufficiently to kill all vegetative organisms; cross-contamination from raw to cooked food in the kitchen must be prevented; and food must be kept at high temperatures or refrigerated so that bacterial multiplication cannot occur. Unpasteurized milk may sometimes be a source of outbreaks, and occasionally salmonella infections spread from person to person directly, but this is very much less important than the route described above.

The predominant symptom is diarrhoea, commencing 1–3 days after ingestion of the food. The disease is benign and self-limiting except at the extremes of age, when a septicaemia may occur. No treatment is usually required. Occasionally, particularly in infants, dehydration may need to be corrected. Antibiotics are not useful and may prolong the period of carriage of the organism.

Diagnosis is by isolation of the organism from the faeces or vomit. Enrichment media such as selenite broth are used. This is subcultured to deoxycholate or MacConkey media. The identification of the non-lactose fermenting organism as a salmonella is made biochemically. Species identification is made on its antigenic structure using antisera to the O antigens and both phases of the H antigens. Species identification is useful for epidemiological purposes and for distinguishing food poisoning salmonellas from the causative agents of enteric fever.

Campylobacter food poisoning

Campylobacter jejuni and *Campylobacter coli* are micro-aerophilic vibrios which are now becoming recognized as important causes of human diarrhoea. The illness may last for a period of about 2 weeks. There are several days' malaise before the onset of diarrhoea, which may be associated with severe abdominal cramps. Campylobacter infections are common in animals, and milk and intensively reared chickens are common sources of infections. The diagnosis is made by the isolation from the faeces of the vibrio using selective media at 43°C under micro-aerophilic conditions.

Staphylococcus aureus food poisoning

This is due to ingestion of pre-formed toxin in the food in which *Staphylococcus aureus* strains have multiplied. The symptoms occur 1–5 hours following ingestion of the food, and vomiting, nausea, and faintness are particularly marked. The illness is short-lived and self-limiting. The sources of the organism are kitchen workers who are symptomless nasal or skin carriers or who have staphylococcal lesions. Prevention is by keeping food too hot or too cold for the organism to multiply, but the toxin once formed is heat resistant and will withstand boiling.

Clostridium perfringens (welchii) food poisoning

Because this anaerobic bacillus is a spore-forming organism, it will frequently survive normal cooking temperatures. Food poisoning is often associated with meat stews, soups and large joints in which anaerobic conditions are found. The disease is caused by the release of an enterotoxin in the bowel as the bacteria sporulate. The symptoms appear 8–24 hours after ingestion of the food and again the condition is benign and self-limiting.

Typical food poisoning strains are non-haemolytic and heat-resistant. The diagnosis may be made by isolating such organisms from the food or the faeces of patients. This may be aided by heating the faeces to 100°C for 30 minutes, when many other bacteria will be killed. However, typical haemolytic strains will also cause food poisoning and in this case the diagnosis can be made by demonstrating increased numbers of the organism in the bowel.

Bacillus cereus food poisoning

This is usually associated with Chinese restaurants, where the organism may multiply in fried rice to produce a toxin. The ingestion of the toxin results in diarrhoea and vomiting of rapid onset.

Vibrio parahaemolyticus food poisoning

This is due to ingestion of the organism in fish which is eaten raw, or in cooked fish in which cross-contamination from raw fish has occurred. Toxin is produced in the bowel and the disease is of rapid onset and short duration.

Botulism

This is due to the ingestion of pre-formed toxin in food. *Clostridium botulinum* is a spore-forming heat-resistant organism and outbreaks of infection are related to inadequate preservation of food, particularly in home canning and bottling and to the distribution of the organism in soil. This disease may be contrasted with staphylococcal food poisoning. *Clostridium botulinum* is much more heat-resistant than *Staphylococcus aureus*, but the toxin produced is heat labile whereas that of *Staphylococcus aureus* will withstand boiling. This affects the conditions under which food poisonign caused by the two organisms occurs. Botulinus toxin is the most potent known and it affects the parasympathetic nervous system producing characteristic signs. Treatment is by antitoxin but the disease is often fatal.

DYSENTERY

This may be bacillary or amoebic.

Bacillary dysentery

The causative agents are the shigellae. In temperate climates *Shigella sonnei* is the commonest pathogen. The symptoms of the disease are abdominal cramps with the passage of stools containing blood and mucus, and the disease can vary from a mild illness to a prolonged, severe, and debilitating one. The disease caused by *Shigella sonnei* is generally mild and that caused by *Shigella dysenteriae* generally severe. However, these distinctions are not clear-cut and *Shigella sonnei* may on occasion cause a severe illness.

Shigella flexneri is also found in temperate climates but less commonly than *Shigella sonnei*. Flexner dysentery is most often seen in vagrants and sometimes in patients in mental hospitals.

Unlike salmonellosis, bacillary dysentery is an exclusively human disease and is spread from man to man via the faecal–oral route.

Contaminated fomites such as lavatory door handles and lavatory seats may be involved. Flies may spread the organism from faeces to food. Outbreaks occur in institutions where it is difficult to maintain high standards of hygiene, such as schools for young children, nurseries, mental hospitals etc., and they may be difficult to control. Outbreaks may occur following a period of warm weather but can continue into the winter months. The disease is diagnosed by isolating the causative organism from the faeces using selective media such as deoxycholate medium. Identification is by the biochemical reactions of the organism, and the antigenic differences between species can be demonstrated serologically. Treatment is supportive but antibiotic therapy may be necessary for the severe forms of the illness.

Amoebic dysentery

Amoebic dysentery is an important disease of world-wide distribution; it is more common in the tropics and sub-tropics than in temperate zones. It is a disease primarily of man and man is the source and reservoir of infection.

The life cycle of *Entamoeba histolytica* is shown in Chapter II. The disease is spread by the cysts via the faecal–oral route. Faecal contamination of water and food is the most important route of infection.

Infecting organism

Entamoeba histolytica is a protozoan of the class Rhizopoda. The trophozoite, which is the active form of the organism, moves with a gliding movement. Cystic forms of the organism are regularly seen; these are smaller, rounded and surrounded by a protective wall.

Clinical features

In the primary lesion the disease is confined to the large bowel. The trophozoites invade the mucosa and sub-mucosa producing ulcers, which are limited by the smooth muscle of the intestinal wall. The presence of these ulcers gives rise to the symptoms of dysentery, that is the passage of stools containing blood and mucus.

The trophozoites may be carried in the portal vein to give rise to an amoebic liver abscess. Amoebic abscesses vary in size but may be very large. Less commonly, metastatic lesions occur in other organs, particularly the lung and brain. The symptoms of amoebic abscesses are related predominantly to the destruction of tissue.

Laboratory diagnosis

This is usually made by the demonstration of the trophozoites in a fresh stool. They can be recognized by their characteristic movement and by the presence of ingested red blood cells. Asymptomatic carriers may be detected by demonstrating the presence of cysts in the stool. It is important to distinguish *Entamoeba histolytica* from non-pathogenic *Entamoeba coli* which may be present.

Amoebic abscesses may be diagnosed by examination of the pus, but if this is not possible, the presence of cysts in the faeces demonstrates amoebic infection, and serological tests, particularly a complement fixation text, are useful.

Prophylaxis

This disease can be prevented by the proper disposal of human faeces so that food and water supplies are not contaminated.

Treatment

A large number of drugs have an action on *Entamoeba histolytica*. Those commonly used now include metronidazole and paromomycin.

GASTRO-ENTERITIS IN INFANTS

This is on a world-wide scale an enormous problem, being particularly important in malnourished children in developing countries. However, even in developed countries gastro-enteritis is a significant cause of morbidity and mortality in infants under the age of 6 months. All the pathogens which affect adults may cause illness in infants, but only those which are important in infants and less significant in adults will be considered here. They are *E. coli* and rotaviruses.

E. coli gastro-enteritis

In developed countries this is seen particularly in units which provide specialist surgical and medical services for babies from a wide area. Although the disease does not appear to be as severe as it was a few years ago, outbreaks still occur. The symptoms are extremely variable and range from the occasional loose stool to severe prolonged watery diarrhoea with rapid dehydration. Prevention of outbreaks of infection can be difficult. Young babies should be nursed individually and infants admitted to a unit from another institution may be barrier nursed until shown to be free from infection.

Any baby with diarrhoea, however mild, should immediately be barrier nursed. Treatment is rehydration if necessary; antibiotics probably have little part to play. Laboratory diagnosis is unsatisfactory. It involves the isolation of strains of *E. coli* with certain 'O' antigens such as 026 or 0111, which are known to cause the condition. The strains of *E. coli* causing infantile gastro-enteritis have not generally been shown to produce toxins or to be entero-invasive as have the strains associated with travellers' diarrhoea.

Viral gastro-enteritis in infants

A number of viruses may be associated with this condition. The most important one is rotavirus. The disease is common in the winter and the infant suffers from diarrhoea and vomiting. The only treatment required may be rehydration and the condition usually resolves in about 4 days. Prevention of spread of infection in a baby unit may be attempted by isolation of affected infants.

TRAVELLERS' DIARRHOEA

Travellers in hot climates, particularly those coming from temperate zones, may suffer from diarrhoea due to any of the pathogens already mentioned. However, many cases are not due to these pathogens, and *E. coli* and some viruses have been considered to be causative agents. These may be carried by the local population and may contaminate food and water.

Strains of *E. coli* which produce enterotoxin or which are entero-invasive have been isolated from cases of travellers' diarrhoea. Among the viruses considered, parvovirus may be important.

ENTERIC FEVER

This is a systemic illness caused by *Salmonella typhi* or *paratyphi* A, B or C, although some strains of *Salmonella paratyphi* may give rise to food poisoning. Unlike other forms of salmonella infection, enteric fever is a human disease and most outbreaks occur when water supplies become contaminated with human excreta, but food and milk-borne outbreaks also occur. Spread of infection in these ways is particularly likely to occur because following an attack of typhoid which may be so mild as to be undiagnosed, intestinal or urinary carriage of the organism may continue for many years. These symptomless excretors may be an important source of infection.

Typhoid fever may be a severe disease, untreated lasting for about 4–5 weeks and symptoms referable to the intestinal tract may be few. During the early part of the illness there is malaise, headache, and fever; this is followed by a period of increasing severity of the illness in which there may be diarrhoea. The severity of the illness diminishes in weeks 3 to 4. Typhoid is a generalized disease, and osteomyelitis, meningitis, and myocarditis may occur. Perforation, haemorrhage or stricture of the intestine may complicate the illness. (Enteric fever is discussed further in Chapter X.)

CHOLERA

Cholera is an important disease of wide distribution. It is endemic in the delta of the Ganges but epidemics occur in India and Pakistan, and the disease has spread to the Middle East and parts of Europe. The El Tor strain is particularly associated with outbreaks in Hong Kong and the Philippines. Spread occurs due to contamination of water supplies with the excreta of cases.

Causative organism

Vibrio cholerae, is a comma shaped gram-negative bacillus. Both the classical strain of *Vibrio cholerae* and the El Tor strain produce an enterotoxin which is responsible for the disease.

Clinical features

The illness occurs most severely in malnourished people living under poor conditions. It is characterized by profuse watery diarrhoea and vomiting and the extremely rapid fluid loss results in circulatory collapse. This fluid loss into the bowel is mediated by the potent enterotoxin produced by the vibrio. This toxin activates adenyl cyclase which raises the intracellular level of cyclic adenosine monophosphate. This in turn causes increased secretion of water and electrolytes into the intestinal lumen.

Laboratory diagnosis

The vibrios may be demonstrated in the characteristic fluid faeces ('rice-water stools'). The motile vibrios may be seen on direct microscopy and the organism may be isolated on selective media, usually TCBS medium (thiosulphate/citrate/bile salt/sucrose).

Prophylaxis

The disease may be prevented by the proper disposal of human excreta so that contamination of food and water supplies does not occur.

Vaccination against the disease has some value and is used not only for travellers to endemic areas but also to attempt to control outbreaks in people living under poor conditions, particularly refugees.

Treatment

Primarily rehydration, but oral tetracycline is useful.

PSEUDO-MEMBRANOUS COLITIS

This may occasionally follow antibiotic usage. Many antibiotics have been associated with the disease but clindamycin is possibly the most important. The disease is due to overgrowth in the bowel of *Clostridium difficile* following destruction of the normal flora. Treatment is cessation of the antibiotic and the use of vancomycin.

PARASITIC INFECTIONS

Many parasites may cause symptoms referable to the bowel. In addition to *Entamoeba histolytica* these include another protozoan, *Giardia lamblia*, which may cause mild diarrhoea and steatorrhoea.

The helminths include threadworms, roundworms, hookworms, whipworms, and tapeworms. Many of these may give rise to diarrhoea and abdominal discomfort. They are mentioned briefly in Chapter I.

CHAPTER IX

Infections of Skin, Soft Tissues, and Bones

COMMON SUPERFICIAL BACTERIAL INFECTIONS

Among the commonest afflictions suffered by man are the simple localized infections of his skin and superficial tissues. The skin in health has a considerable normal flora, which includes as permanent residents a variety of micrococci and diphtheroids and in a proportion of people *Staphylococcus aureus*. In addition, many organisms are found more transitorily on the skin, including coliforms, proteus, clostridia, and other bowel organisms which occur most frequently on skin sites near the anus such as the perineum, buttocks, and thighs. Any break in the skin, however minor, whether accidental or by intention in surgery, can be infected by these organisms and of course by others such as streptococci which may be introduced to the tissues.

Furuncles

Boils are due to infection of a hair follicle or sebaceous duct with *Staphylococcus aureus*. They usually affect the hair follicles at the back of the neck, in the axilla or on the face. There is rapid inflammation, swelling, pus formation and necrosis. The centre of the lesion breaks down, the pus and finally the necrotic centre is discharged and healing follows. Local treatment is generally sufficient and it may be helpful to use chlorhexidine soap for washing. Recurrent boils should raise the question of general health and possible diabetes.

Carbuncles

Occasionally the initial staphylococcal folliculitis and furunculosis may become more widely and deeply spread, involving numerous hair follicles and the formation of a considerable abscess. This occurs most often in those with diminished resistance such as in diabetes. The lesion discharges from many follicles but is slow to resolve and surgical interference and therapy with flucloxacillin may be necessary.

Impetigo contagiosa

This superficial infection may be caused by *Staphylococcus aureus* or can be initiated by an infection with *Streptococcus pyogenes* (Group A) and both organisms may be found on culture. Characteristically there is the formation of a small vesicle, which progresses to the discharge of pus which dries in crusts on the skin. The face is almost always the part affected. It is extremely contagious, especially among children, and local treatment with application of chlorhexidine after removal of the crusts should be initiated as soon as possible. If the disease is clearly streptococcal it may be advisable to treat it systemically with penicillin to avoid the danger of nephritis following infection with certain streptococcal strains.

Pemphigus neonatorum is a form of bullous impetigo which is due to *Staphylococcus aureus* generally of phage type 71 (Chapter II). It occurs in outbreaks in nurseries. The same staphylococcal group is found, producing an epidermolytic toxin which causes acute epidermal necrolysis in which large sheets of skin are denuded on the surface of bullae. This usually occurs in children and rarely in adults. These conditions should be treated by flucloxacillin systemically as well as in acute epidermal necrolysis by replacement of lost fluid.

Acne vulgaris

This very distressing and common disorder affects a large proportion of young peole in their teens and may also occur in older people. Sebaceous follicles become blocked and form a blackhead or comedo. Subsequent development is not fully explained but there is inflammation and pus formation in the blocked follicle. Probably the normal commensal flora, particularly *Propionibacterium acnes*, in association with the changed skin conditions after puberty, plays a part in the production of the lesions. These may progress to cystic and pustular acne with severe scarring and keloid formation. Whatever the cause, long term oral tetracycline or erythromycin does have a beneficial effect certainly on pustular acne.

Erysipelas

This superficial infection is due to *Streptococcus pyogenes* (Group A) and appears as a cellulitis of the face or occasionally elsewhere on the body. It is painful, red, sharply defined and affects only the skin and the lymphatics. It is uncommon and can be treated using penicillin or erythromycin.

Other Localized Abscesses

Sepsis following minor trauma can develop in any site but is common in the hands and fingers. It is almost entirely caused by *Staphylococcus aureus*. Paronychia is infection of the nailbed and whitlow is the term used to describe an abscess in the pulp of the finger. Herpetic whitlow due to the herpes simplex virus occurs most often in nurses infected from their patients.

SUPERFICIAL FUNGAL INFECTIONS

The superficial mycoses are caused by infection of the keratinized layers of the skin, hair, and nails by a group of fungi collectively known as the dermatophytes. Candidal infection can also occur affecting those areas of skin in contact and rubbing together such as the perineum and may also affect the nails and nailbeds.

The dermatophytes are of three genera, the Microsporum, Epidermophyton and Trichophyton. Infection is usually from human contagion but may be from animals, e.g. *M. canis*. These superficial fungal infections are usually referred to as Tinea.

Tinea capitis

This infection of the hair on the head may be due to a wide variety of members of the genera microsporum or trichophyton. *M. canis* and *M. audouinii* and *T. tonsurans* are frequent causative agents.

Microsporum infections usually occur in primary schoolchildren, especially in boys. On microscopic examination the fungal spores can be seen to surround the hairs on the outside (ectothrix) and the hairs break off leaving a circular area of scalp with stumps of hair. The hairs fluoresce in UV light.

Trichophyton infections can occur in children and in adults. *T. tonsurans* causes an infection within the hair shaft (endothrix) and when the hairs break off they do so at the surface of the scalp. *T. schoenleinii* causes a chronic crusting infection leading to permanent baldness. The hairs do not fluoresce in UV light in these infections. Treatment of tinea capitis is by oral griseofulvin over a period of 2 months.

Tinea corporis

This fungal infection of the skin is caused by a wide variety of species of Microsporum, Trichophyton and Epidermophyton genera. *M. audouinii* and *M. canis* are often involved as are *T. rubrum*, *T. mentagraphytes* and *E. floccosum*, especially in tinea cruris and tinea unguium. Tinea pedis is most frequently caused by *T. mentagrophytes*.

The typical lesion in tinea corporis is a spreading ring with active vesicles on its outer edge and a healing scaly centre. Tina pedis is usually characterized by inflammation and the formation of fissures. Treatment is generally topical using 1% clotrimazole, or 2% miconazole cream. These applications should be continued twice daily until 2 weeks after the lesions have healed.

Superficial Candidal Infection

This can affect the nails and nailbeds. It is treated by application of nystatin cream or clotrimazole. It is important to continue application 2 weeks after healing. Nappy rash due to candidiasis can be treated by these agents as creams or as dusting powder.

Diagnosis of Superficial Mycosis

Scrapings from the lesions, or pieces of hair, can be examined after treatment with 30% KOH microscopically using the low power objective. The organisms will be seen in hair as spores either surrounding the hair (ectothrix) or within it (endothrix). In skin scrapings broken fragments of hyphae can be seen. In either case identification of the fungus is by culture on Sabouraud's agar for 2 weeks at room temperature.

Colonial appearances and the production of macroconidia are the basis of differentiation (Chapter II).

OTHER SUPERFICIAL INFECTIONS

Cutaneous Anthrax

Bacillus anthracis is the causative organism of anthrax. It is a large Gram-positive rod, aerobic, non-motile, and has an oval central spore.

Anthrax is a disease of animals, especially cattle, horses, sheep, and goats, who ingest the hardy spores of *Bacillus anthracis* from the soil. Enteritis is followed by septicaemia and the outcome is generally fatal.

Man is normally infected directly from infectious animals or carcases, from hides, hair or bone meal. Anthrax may occur in the intestine from ingestion or in the lung from inhalation. Cutaneous anthrax results generally from handling and carrying infected hides or hair. Common sites of the lesion are the hands, arms, and the side of the face, where the organism probably gains access through some minor cut or abrasion. A little red macule forms and becomes vesicular and oedamatous breaking down to form a necrotic ulcer with a characteristic black eschar, the 'Malignant Pustule'. There can be considerable swelling and regional lymphadenitis but the lesion itself is painless.

The organism can sometimes be demonstrated in material from the vesicle or ulcer, and culture may yield large, greyish, usually non-haemolytic colonies on aerobic incubation. Identification is by demonstrating the lytic effect of specific phage.

Active immunization against anthrax is available for all whose work puts them at risk and this together with strict regulations on imported goat hair has reduced the disease to a rarity in Britain.

Treatment is by penicillin in large doses for up to 2 weeks and is usually successful.

Actinomycosis

The causative organism in man is a Gram-positive, filamentous branching bacterium, *Actinomyces israelii*. Most strains are anaerobic but micro-aerophilic strains occur and CO_2 may assist growth. It exists in the mouth as a commensal and invades the tissues following trauma or dental treatment. It can also be inhaled or swallowed.

The usual lesion is a chronic slowly enlarging swelling of the face or jaw although it may develop more acutely. There may be suppuration and the formation of fistulas. Pus may contain the characteristic 'sulphur granules' which are tangled masses of the filamentous mycelia. Crushed on a microscope slide the Gram-negative clubs round the edge of the granule can also be seen. Modified Ziehl–Neelsen staining using 1% H_2SO_4 for decolorization shows the clubs are acid fast. The organism can be cultivated anaerobically in broth or blood agar. Treatment is by penicillin for 2 months but surgical drainage may also be necessary.

Herpes simplex

This virus can produce a variety of clinical conditions. Genital herpes is considered in Chapter VII and acute necrotizing encephalitis in Chapter V.

The virus attacks most people at some time in life, generally sub-clinically. Pre-school children may suffer vesicular lesions on the mucous membrane of the mouth and gums or occasionally conjunctivitis (Chapter III). With increasing age there is a steady rise in the number of people showing evidence of antibody production.

The common superficial infection is the 'cold sore', an eruption of vesicles around the mouth and nose. This is recurrent due to the ability of the virus to lie dormant in the sensory nerve cells of the host. Fresh lesions erupt apparently due to unrelated stimuli and eradication is very difficult. The antiviral agent idoxuridine can be applied to the lesions but is not very effective.

INFECTIONS OF BONE

Acute Pyogenic Osteomyelitis

This infection may affect any bone and can occur at any age. It most commonly attacks the long bones of children, involving the metaphyses close to the actively growing epiphyses. It nearly always is due to *Staphylococcus aureus*, although occasionally other organisms are involved.

It usually arises as a blood-borne infection and a pre-disposing factor is local trauma. It can also occur as a complication of a compound fracture or sometimes by direct spread of an abscess into the bone, particularly in the jaw.

Once established in the cancellous bone the infection can spread to involve adjacent tissues, particularly the periosteum, and may progress to thrombosis of the blood supply, necrosis of the bone and the formation of sequestra. There may be invasion of the bloodstream, septicaemia and death. The disease may also not resolve and may end as chronic osteomyelitis with recurrent discharge of pus from sinuses. All these conditions are rarely seen now in developed countries since the introduction of antibiotics.

Diagnosis is on clinical and radiographic grounds but the organism may often be found on blood culture in the early stages and of course in discharged pus or in a needle biopsy.

Treatment is dependent on the antibiotic sensitivity of the organism.

In staphylococcal infection penicillin should be combined with cloxacillin or fucidin until the sensitivity is known and then the appropriate agent continued for 3 weeks. Surgical drainage or open surgery may be necessary. Haemophilus osteomyelitis is best treated with ampicillin. Osteomyelitis can occur rarely in salmonella infections and brucellosis and is sometimes caused by anaerobic organisms and Gram-negative bacilli including *Pseudomonas aeruginosa*.

Tuberculosis of Bone

This condition is uncommon in countries in which bovine tuberculosis has been eradicated. Now it is due to human strains of *M. tuberculosis* which spread from existing lesions of the lung or other organisms via the bloodstream. Most commonly affected are the vertebrae (Pott's Disease) and the femur and tibia near the hip and knee.

The infection starts as osteomyelitis with inflammation, the formation of granulation tissues and then erosion and necrosis of bone. In the spine the destruction leads to collapse of the vertebrae and the development of deformities and possibly paraplegia. The whole process is slow and often insidious. There may be spread of pus from the spine along tissue planes to form cold abscesses. Eventual healing is by fibrosis. Laboratory diagnosis may be difficult but the organism may be grown from the discharge from sinuses or abscesses or from biopsy specimens and its demonstration in sputum or urine may be a helpful pointer and enable its sensitivity to anti-tuberculous drugs to be determined. Treatment with appropriate agents should be continued for 18 months.

GAS GANGRENE

This very serious infection is caused by *Clostridium perfringens* or occasionally by *Clostridium oedematiens* or *Clostridium septicum*. These are anaerobic sporing organisms which are part of the normal intestinal flora of man and animals. Their spores survive well in soil and dust and are widespread in the environment. They may be introduced into a wound either at the time of trauma in a traffic accident or in war or in the course of surgery, particularly involving the bowel or areas contaminated by organisms from it. They find favourable conditions to germinate, multiply, and establish themselves where there is little or no oxygen due to damaged or deficient circulation following injury or in vascular insufficiency due to obliterative disease. Foreign bodies, dead tissue, and the presence of other pyogenic organisms are contributing factors favourable to the development of the clostridia.

Once established the clostridia attack the body tissues with a wide variety of exotoxins including lecithinase and hyaluronidase which lyse and destroy cells and their membranes. A swollen, oedematous painful lesion develops. The production of gas during the putrefaction and fermentation gives rise to the characteristic crepitation due to the bubbles in the tissues. There is acute haemolysis which may lead to renal failure. Death occurs due to toxaemia.

Laboratory diagnosis is by examination of swabs, tissue fluids, or tissue from the affected area when the large Gram-positive bacilli may be seen often in mixed culture. Culture anaerobically on blood agar or in Robertson's Cooked Meat Broth gives a growth which can be identified by demonstrating the Nagler reaction.

It is important to realize that growth of *Clostridium perfringens* from a wound does not mean that there is gas gangrene. The organism is a common contaminant of the skin especially in the perineum, hip, buttocks and thighs and may be found in the absence of gangrene. Treatment of gas gangrene is by surgical debridement of all dead tissue and the removal of foreign bodies, together with antibiotic therapy with very large doses of penicillin. Hyperbaric oxygen is now of proven value but antitoxin does not seem to influence the outcome. Prophylactic antibiotic therapy is essential in surgery involving amputation, in obliterative vascular conditions or in orthopaedic surgery on the hip joint or neck of femur. Penicillin must be given to cover the period of the operation.

TETANUS

This disease is caused by the action of the neurotoxin tetanospasmin produced by *Clostridium tetani* after it has established itself in the body. The organism, an anaerobic spore bearing, motile, slender, Gram-positive rod is found with varying frequency as part of the faecal flora of animals and sometimes man. Its spores are highly resistant to heat and drying and are widespread in dust and soil. Classically tetanus follows deep severe penetrating wounds but can also follow small or insignificant wounds and because of their greater frequency most tetanus is seen following such minor trauma. Development of the disease is favoured by anaerobic conditions and poor circulation and foreign bodies in the wound. Germination of the spores is followed by multiplication and then elaboration of the neurotoxin. The toxin travels up the motor nerves either directly from the site of the wound or after circulation in the bloodstream, via motor nerves generally and reaches the central nervous system. Clinical disease follows within a few days in central wounds and up to 3 weeks in peripheral wounds. There is spasm of the jaw, stiffness of the neck and spasm of the back muscles, progressing to generalized tetanic seizures. Mortality in untreated cases is very high but with intensive care recovery occurs in almost all cases. Diagnosis is on clinical grounds. The organism often cannot be demonstrated microscopically or cultured from the wound which may only be a minor abrasion. If seen it has a characteristic drumstick appearance. Culture must be strictly anaerobic usually on blood agar or in Robertson's cooked meat broth.

Treatment of tetanus once established is largely a matter of controlling the spasms until the disease resolves and preventing the production of further toxin by the *Clostridium tetani* in the wound. Penicillin should be given, the wound cleaned and excised if necessary. Tetanus antitoxin may be given although it has no effect on toxin already in the nervous system and human anti tetanus immunoglobulin must be chosen as it is much less liable to cause allergic or anaphylactic reactions. Control of the spasms requires sedation and relaxation with chlorpromazine or other sedatives. In the most serious uncontrollable spasms this should be used together with paralysis of the voluntary muscles by curare and artificial ventilation through a tracheostomy. In this situation the greatest danger to the patient lies in nosocomial infection.

Immunization against tetanus is safe and effective and this is now a totally preventable disease. It should be remembered that many cases of tetanus occur in wounds of such minor nature that no special regimen and often no treatment at all seems to be indicated. For this reason active immunization should be encouraged for the whole population but especially for those particularly at risk such as gardeners, farmers and those in the armed forces. Should a person fully immunized receive a wound thought liable to be infected by *Clostridium tetani* all that is necessary is a full wound cleansing and a booster dose of tetanus toxoid. Antibiotic cover may also be advisable for 10 days. An unimmunized person presents a more difficult problem although the advent of Human Tetanus Immunoglobulin (HTI) has removed the greatest risk of anaphylactic shock which prevented the use of horse anti-tetanic serum to give immediate passive protection. HTI should now be given together with a complete course of tetanus toxoid to give immediate passive protection and then long lasting active immunity.

CHAPTER X

Generalized Bacterial, Spirochaetal, and Rickettsial Infections

This chapter considers a number of important infections which affect the body generally rather than invade just a single organ. Some other infections include as part of the disease process a brief generalized invasion either in the early stages or as a late complication or terminal event, but they are characterized by a particular selective effect on one organ or system and are discussed in the appropriate chapter.

GENERALIZED BACTERIAL INFECTIONS

Septicaemia

There is a distinction between 'bacteraemia', in which organisms temporarily gain access to the blood stream from some port of entry or some disease focus, and 'septicaemia', in which the organisms overcome the defences of the host, invade the blood stream and multiply within it. This can produce severe toxaemia which may damage the vascular system and the major organs and there is often the establishment of multiple small septic foci throughout the body. Septicaemia can be due to any pathogenic organism but is commonly caused by only a few.

Staphylococcal septicaemia

Staphylococcal lesions (Chapter IX) are generally localized, for example as boils, or septic wounds, or osteomyelitis, and do not usually invade the body generally. Such invasion does sometimes occur and is particularly likely when the defences of the host are compromised in the old and the very young and the immunologically deficient. The patient becomes febrile with rigors, sweating, and confusion and may go into coma and die. Blood culture is positive and sensitivity testing is a guide to antibiotic therapy. This is usually with cloxacillin and gentamicin intravenously.

Gram-negative septicaemia

Generalized invasion of the blood stream with Gram-negative bacilli is a growing problem, particularly in patients with diminished resistance and those on antibiotic therapy. The organisms most often involved include *Escherichia coli*, klebsiella and *Pseudomonas aeruginosa*, while proteus spp., other enterobacteriaceae and serratia are also found. Factors predisposing to septicaemia with Gram-negative bacilli are surgical interference with the intestinal or genito-urinary tract. *Pseudomonas aeruginosa* is particularly associated with hospitalization and antibiotic therapy, when it increasingly colonizes the patient and can give rise to especially serious invasions very resistant to antibiotic treatment.

In Gram-negative rod septicaemia the pyrexia, rigors, and malaise are often complicated by 'endotoxic' or 'septic' shock in which there is hypotension and oliguria. This appears to be associated with the production of endotoxins by the bacilli.

Antibiotic therapy should be begun empirically with gentamicin and altered if necessary following the results of blood culture and sensitivity testing. It is important to maintain cardiac output and electrolyte balance in patients with septic shock.

Anaerobic septicaemia

This is almost always due to *Bacteroides fragilis*, the common anaerobe of the lower bowel, and usually follows serious surgery or disease of the intestine or genito-urinary tract. The organism is a delicate Gram-negative bacillus less strictly anaerobic than most of the other bacteroides, but which grows best anaerobically in 10% CO_2. If diagnosed by blood culture or if strongly suspected, treatment should be instituted with metronidazole. Clindamycin may be used but sometimes gives rise to pseudomembranous colitis.

Other septicaemia

Many organisms can cause septicaemia in suitable conditions. Group B streptococci are particularly important in neonates (see Chapter V). *Neisseria meningitidis* may cause acute fulminating septicaemia with skin rashes, collapse and death from necrosis of the adrenal glands, the Waterhouse–Friderichsen syndrome.

Streptococcus pneumoniae and *Haemophilus influenzae* are also organisms which may be involved. Organisms such as the salmonellae and *Yersinia pestis* are considered below. Patients with septicaemia must be treated rapidly, often before the causative organism is known. Gentamicin must be given and can be accompanied by metronidazole if there is any indication of likely anaerobic involvement and amoxycillin if there is not.

Rheumatic Fever

This disease follows 2 to 3 weeks after a streptococcal throat infection in a small percentage of patients, usually schoolchildren and young people. It is characterized by inflammation of connective tissue, particularly in the heart, where it affects the endocardium and also the myocardium and pericardium.

Why this occurs is not fully understood but auto-immunity would seem to play a part with the tissues of the heart damaged following attachment of some cross-reacting antibody to streptococcal antigen. Acute myocarditis and pericarditis may occur and be fatal. Acute endocarditis also occurs and on the heart valves can give rise to the formation of thrombi or vegetations. Recurrences are frequent and the disease may progress to chronic rheumatic heart disease affecting the myocardium and the valves. Rheumatic heart disease predisposes to bacterial endocarditis.

It is important that streptococcal infections especially in young people are treated by adequate antibiotic therapy to prevent the occurrence of rheumatic fever. Patients with rheumatic fever should be kept clear of subsequent streptococcal infection by long term oral penicillin (see under Bacterial Endocarditis).

Bacterial Endocarditis

This is an infection of the endocardium typically giving rise to the formation of masses or vegetations on its surface. Often the site of attachment of these crumbling masses is where there is pre-existent abnormality or damage. Heart valves damaged by rheumatic fever or congenital abnormality or valvular impants and prostheses are commonly affected.

The infecting organisms are often not clearly recognized pathogens but are regarded as commensals of the body and are acting as opportunists. The most common of these agents is *Streptococcus viridans*, a commensal of the respiratory tract. *Streptococcus faecalis*, a common organism of the bowel, and *Staphylococcus epidermidis*, a commensal of the skin are also found. Occasionally candida, other fungi and Gram-negative bacilli may be involved. Endocarditis due to *Staphylococcus aureus* may follow cardiac surgery or haemodialysis.

The development of infection is often insidious, depending on a sub-clinical transient bacteraemia accompanying dental treatment or as little trauma as teeth-scaling or even grinding of the teeth. Interference with the urinary tract such as catheterization or any other surgery can release Gram-negative bacilli and enterococci into the blood stream. More directly, vascular or cardiac surgery may do so, as well as providing a suitable site for the establishment of the infection. In any case the circulating organisms adhere to and colonize the damaged endocardium forming the characteristic vegetations. Subsequently there is a continuing low grade infection with intermittent bacteraemia and discharge of emboli, fever and splenomegaly. Death was inevitable in the untreated patient.

Diagnosis is by demonstrating the causative organism in blood culture.

Treatment

Prophylaxis

Prevention of the establishment of bacterial endocarditis is of paramount importance and the chain of events which can lead to it, from streptococcal infection to rheumatic fever and then to endocarditis, must be interrupted by antibiotic therapy. Antibiotic treatment of streptococcal infection has been a major contribution, reducing the incidence of rheumatic fever. Patients who do develop rheumatic fever may receive long term prophylaxis using penicillin to prevent recurrences with consequent damage to the heart valves. Patients in whom the heart valves have been damaged, or patients with congenital defects or cardiac prostheses, should be offered prophylactic antibiotic cover when dental or surgical interference is taking place and such interference should be carried out only if absolutely necessary.

In dentistry or tonsillectomy, cover is given by oral penicillin with benzyl penicillin or amoxycillin orally in a single dose just before the operation. If the patient is already receiving penicillin as prophylaxis for rheumatic fever another agent such as erythromycin must be substituted as the patient's own oral commensal streptococci will be resistant.

Operations on sites likely to give rise to bacteraemia with *Streptococcus faecalis* or Gram-negative bacilli can be covered using gentamicin with ampicillin. Cardiac surgery can be covered with gentamicin and cloxacillin although other regimens may be chosen. It may be necessary to change the prophylactic regimen advocated in a cardiac surgery unit from time to time to help to prevent the establishment of antibiotic resistant organisms.

Therapy

Treatment of established bacterial endocarditis depends on which organism is responsible and requires extensive laboratory assistance to ensure that there are bactericidal levels of antibiotics (Chapter XVI). The most commonly involved organism, *Streptococcus viridans*, is usually relatively sensitive to benzyl penicillin although this does vary. *Streptococcus faecalis* is relatively resistant to penicillin and the staphylococci both aureus and epidermidis are usually resistant. Streptococcal endocarditis then should be treated using benzyl penicillin with gentamicin although amoxycillin and gentamicin may be preferred. Staphylococcal endocarditis requires the use of cloxacillin and gentamicin. These regimens have to be continued for several weeks at least. Alternative treatment may be dictated by developing allergy or by the occasional superinfection of the valve by resistant organisms.

Enteric Fever

Enteric fever includes typhoid caused by *Salmonella typhi* and paratyphoid caused by *Salmonella paratyphi* A, B, or C. These salmonellae are members of a genus belonging to the enterobacteriaeceae family. Within the genus are more than 1700 distinguishable serotypes. The organisms of enteric fever can be distinguished from the large numbers of others in the genus in that they are human pathogens which do not normally affect animals, whereas the vast majority of salmonellae are animal parasites although they do infect man. Another major practical distinction is that the enteric fever organisms typically cause a general systemic infection whereas the others usually cause a simple food poisoning by their invasion of the gastro-intestinal tract, although they can on occasion cause systemic infection particularly in hosts with reduced resistance due to age, disease, or other factors.

Typhoid

Pathology

The ingested organisms first multiply in the lymph nodes draining the small bowel and then pass to the blood stream and are widely disseminated throughout the organs of the body including the spleen, kidney, liver, gall bladder, heart and bone marrow. Probably from the gall bladder there is subsequently further invasion of the intestine with multiplication in the lymphoid tissue, inflammation, necrosis and sloughing leading to the formation of typhoid ulcers.

Clinical features

The organism is ingested in water or food contaminated by a human excretor. The incubation period varies from 7 to 21 days but is usually 10–14 days. It is influenced by the dose of organisms ingested, being shorter with heavier doses. Onset is insidious with headache, fever, general pains, apathy, and sometimes epistaxis. Constipation is usual and diarrhoea less common. Characteristically the pulse rate is slow in proportion to the temperature. The characteristic rash consisting of 'rose spots' appears after 7–10 days and affects the trunk. The spleen is usually enlarged and there may be meningism. The 'pea soup' stool is by no means always found. Leucopenia is a characteristic sign.

Laboratory diagnosis

This can be divided into three phases.

1) *Salmonella typhi* can be cultured from the blood in the first week and blood cultures may often remain positive for 2–3 weeks thereafter. Success can sometimes be obtained by culturing the clot from blood specimens after removal of the patient's serum which may contain inhibitory antibodies.

2) Culture of *Salmonella typhi* from faeces is generally positive during the second and third weeks of illness, but may be positive before and after that time. Culture of urine may also yield positive results in the second and third weeks in some cases. Further epidemiological information may be obtained by phage typing the organisms.

3) Demonstration of antibodies to *Salmonella typhi* in the patient's serum is the basis of the Widal Test, in which agglutinating antibodies to the O, H, and Vi antigens of *Salmonella typhi* are sought usually together with the antibodies to *Salmonella paratyphi* B, O, and H antigens (Chapter XIX). The interpretation of positive results is not easy. Agglutination indicates some exposure to the antigen at some time. A rising titre indicates that the antibody level is being increased either by active disease or some other non-specific stimulus. TAB inoculation (Chapter XVIII) can give considerable titres and the H antibodies can

persist for some years. Vi antibody may also help in indicating the possibility that an individual is a carrier of typhoid (see below) although Vi titres are found in non-carriers also. The Vi antigen may protect the organism against phagocytosis and thus contribute to enhanced virulence.

In a simple uncomplicated case O and H antibody titres to *Salmonella typhi* would be expected reaching 1/40 to 1/80 within a week, subsequently going to much higher levels. Rising titres are particularly significant. In previously protected patients, TAB inoculation may give high and rising titres and interpretation is especially difficult. Vi titres may be 1/5 in many normal people and they should be interpreted with exceptional care.

Treatment

The drug of choice for many years now has been chloramphenicol orally for 2 weeks. It is the most effective antibiotic but has two disadvantages. Resistance to it is increasingly emerging and it has to be used in awareness or its rare but fatal side effect of aplastic anaemia. Relapses can follow treatment. Many other agents have been used in treatment including cotrimoxazole and ampicillin. They are no more effective than chloramphenicol but may be preferred particularly in mild cases because of the dangers of chloramphenicol.

Carriage of Salmonella typhi

All patients with clinical typhoid and the few who are infected subclinically excrete the organism in their faeces and sometimes in their urine for a period of some weeks. After 3 months only a small percentage still do so and at this point they may be described as carriers. Faecal carriage is much the more common and the gall bladder and hepatic ducts are the site of the focus of infection. Pre-existing disease of the gall bladder or the presence of gallstones may predispose to the carrier state. Renal carriers, though rarer, do occur and again the presence of pre-existing disease is an important factor. It should be remembered in detection of carriage by culture of stools or urine that excretion can be intermittent. Treatment of carriers is extremely difficult and even prolonged therapy with ampicillin in high dosage may not be successful. Surgical interference by cholecystectomy or removal of gallstones or by removal of an abnormal or diseased kidney can be effective in some cases.

Paratyphoid

This infection is due to *Salmonella paratyphi* A, B, or C, with different serotypes occurring more commonly in different parts of the world. In Western Europe *Salmonella paratyphi* B is most common but A is found widely elsewhere and C in the Far East.

On the whole, but not invariably, paratyphoid is a less serious infection than typhoid. It is an infection of man rather than animals and while it produces the classical systemic infection of enteric fever it often causes only an enteritis. The incidence of complications and relapses is lower than in typhoid and the mortality rate is very low. Treatment of paratyphoid is the same as that of typhoid.

Brucellosis

This is a disease of animals due to infection with species of the genus *Brucella*. Man is infected by direct contact with the animals or by drinking their infected milk.

Infecting organisms

Three species are important in human disease:
Brucella melitensis —associated with sheep and goats but may affect cattle and pigs occasionslly;
Brucella abortus —associated with cattle and occasionally with sheep and pigs;
Brucella suis —associated with pigs but may affect sheep.
All are Gram-negative, cocco-bacilli, 0.5–0.7 by 0.6–1.5μ, non-motile and aerobic. *Brucella abortus* grows better in the presence of 5% CO_2. The species can be identified by their growth on media containing basic fuschin or thionin dyes. There are a number of biotypes within all these species and there is very considerable antigenic variation among the biotypes as well as considerable similarity among the species.

Clinical features

The disease is one of veterinarians, farmers and abattoir workers who may have no choice but to have close contact with diseased animals, but regrettably is still also a disease of those who drink raw milk or milk products from diseased cows or goats. Brucellosis eradication programmes among cattle and pasteurization of milk can reduce the incidence to a very low level, but the infection is still rife in many countries. The disease is not spread from man to man. The organism is usually ingested, although in occupational brucellosis inhalation is probable. Incubation periods vary from weeks to months, but once established the disease presents acutely or more insidiously as a pyrexial illness with aches and pains, very profuse sweating, and chills. Unfortunately very often the diagnosis is not made at this point and the patient proceeds to a sub-acute phase, with tiredness, aches and pains, depression, and fluctuating bouts of pyrexia. Chronic brucellosis may follow in a few patients with continued low grade symptoms, or a wide variety of complications can occur including arthritis, osteomyelitis, endocarditis, and epididymitis.

Laboratory diagnosis

In the acute phase a high index of suspicion may lead to investigation by blood culture. Incubation should be continued for up to 6 weeks and the presence of 5% CO_2 enhances growth of *Brucella abortus* strains. At this stage there is a fall in the number of polymorphonuclear leucocytes. Culture of the organism in the early stages is easy but it can readily cause serious laboratory infection and must be handled circumspectly. In many cases culture is attempted too late and often diagnosis in the later stages depends on serology. In the acute phase of the disease IgM antibodies are produced in abundance together with some IgG antibodies. Normally with recovery both antibodies fall and disappear, although it may still be possible to detect low levels of IgM for some time. If the disease remains active, IgG antibody remains in the serum. IgA antibody is also produced and is responsible for skin sensitivity to Brucella antigen. A number of tests are available to demonstrate and differentiate between these antibodies.

1) Direct agglutination test

This depends on IgM antibody agglutinating a prepared suspension of brucella organisms.

2) Indirect agglutination test (anti-human globulin)

This depends on IgG antibody binding to the organisms without agglutinating them. After washing away all IgG antibodies not bound to the organisms, the addition of anti-human globulin to the suspension will bind with the IgG human globulin and give visible clumping of the organisms.

3) Complement fixation test

Reaction between IgG antibody and the brucella organism fixes complement and can be used to demonstrate the presence of this antibody.

The interpretation of these tests is not straightforward and the results have to be considered carefully together with the whole clinical picture. Table X.1 shows some expected findings.

Table X.1

Test	Antibodies	Acute <3 months	Sub-acute <1 year	Chronic 1–35 years
Direct agglutination	IgM 19 S macro-globulin	+ + + Rising titre	+ +	± →0
Anti-human globulin test	(IgA) IgG 7 S micro-globulin	+	+ +	+ + +
Complement Fixation test	IgG 7 S micro-globulin	+	+	+

In the acute phase a rising titre is more clearly indicative of brucellosis than a single titre of 1/80. Levels may rise to 1/640 or 1/1280 in 2–3 weeks.

There is very considerable overlap in serological titres between species of brucella.

Treatment

Tetracycline with streptomycin for the first 3 weeks followed by tetracycline alone reduces bacteraemia in the acute phase and the frequency of relapse. Cotrimoxazole is a useful alternative and should be given for up to 2 months.

Plague

This disease, which is not now seen in Europe, was once one of the great scourges of mankind, wiping out large numbers of the population in devastating epidemics. It is still endemic in large areas of Asia and occurs in Africa and America. It is caused by infection with *Yersinia pestis*, a small non-motile, Gram-negative bacillus, which is sometimes capsulated and which shows typical bipolar staining when stained by methylene blue. The yersinia are a genus of the family enterobacteriaeceae and include *Yersinia pseudotuberculosis* and *Yersinia enterocolitica*.

Bubonic plague

Normally enzootic in rodents, bubonic plague is carried to humans by the bite of the rate flea *Xenopsylla cheopsis*, usually from *Rattus rattus* the house rat. It can occasionally arise among those such as trappers in contact with wild rodents. Depending on the site of the flea bite a 'bubo' develops usually in the axilla, groin, or neck within 24 hours. This consists of swelling and enlargement of the lymph nodes with haemorrhage and necrosis. Septicaemia follows and death in many cases.

Pneumonic plague

This disease is passed from rodent to person in inhaled dust and subsequently by droplet inhalation from person to person. It is a serious acute pneumonia with a high mortality. Diagnosis is by demonstrating the organism in the sputum. It may also be present in the blood in the septicaemic phase. Treatment is by streptomycin and chloramphenicol or cotrimoxazole. Prevention depends on control of rats and eradication of fleas. Immunization is of some value but any protection is unfortunately shortlived.

Leprosy

This infection still affects millions of people in tropical regions and may be found in occasional immigrants to other areas. It is due to infection with *Mycobacterium leprae*, a straight or slightly curved rod, long and strongly acid fast. The disease is described as taking two main forms, 'tuberculoid', which occurs in patients with relatively high immunity and which is a more limited form of the disease, and 'lepromatous', which occurs in those with less immunity and which is more generalized. There is a whole range of clinical conditions between these and the disease may vary in its nature in an individual patient as time passes.

Tuberculoid leprosy is characterized by skin lesions which appear as large plaques with raised edges and a flattened centre. There is hair loss from the plaque and it is anaesthetic. Nerve damage is usually of limited distribution. The organisms are never more than scanty in these lesions.

Lepromatous leprosy usually presents as multiple lesions, nodular or papular. The face is often affected, with thickening of the skin giving 'leonine facies', loss of eyebrows and later destruction of the nasal cartilages. The lesions are packed with bacilli and large macrophages. Nerve involvement is more patchy with 'glove' or 'stocking' anaesthesia.

Diagnosis in the laboratory consists of demonstrating the organisms in scrapings or biopsies. They cannot be cultured in vitro but are cultivated in the foot pads of immunologically compromised mice or in the armadillo.

Treatment is by dapsone for several years or even indefinitely. Rifampicin should also be given for the first 6 months of treatment in lepromatous leprosy. Dapsone resistance is a developing problem and clofazimine may be useful in these circumstances.

GENERALIZED SPIROCHAETAL INFECTIONS

Leptospirosis

The leptospira are a genus of the spirochaetaceae family which includes in other genera the treponemes and the borrelia. There are two species complexes: *Leptospira interrogans* which contains those serotypes which are pathogenic in man, including *Leptospira icterohaemorrhagiae* and *Leptospira canicola*; and the *Leptospira biflexa* complex whose members are generally saprophytic. Leptospirosis is a disease which affects a wide variety of animals including rats, dogs, cattle, and pigs. Man is infected when the spirochaete enters through a minor break in his skin or by the mucous membrane usually of mouth or conjunctiva. This may follow direct contact with the animal or be from contamination by the animal's urine. The disease does not normally spread from person to person. It is commoner in those working in sewers, old mines, and farmyards where rats abound, but is found also in anglers and those enjoying swimming or water sports in rivers and ponds.

The infecting organism

The leptospire is a slender spirochaete with tight coils. Characteristically it is hooked at one or both ends and is freely motile with a variety of active movements. It can be cultured in fluid media containing rabbit serum, aerobically at 30°C.

Clinical features

The incubation period after the organism has entered the body is usually 7–10 days, after which there is a septicaemic phase in which there may be a high temperature, headache, severe myalgia, conjunctivitis, and prostration. The organism affects all organs and can be found in the blood and the CSF. The liver and the kidney may both be affected and there may be jaundice and renal failure. Weil's disease, which is an acute severe infection with jaundice, haematuria and vascular collapse, has still a mortality of 10%. It is generally caused by *Leptospira icterohaemor-rhagiae*. *Leptospira canicola* infections are usually less severe and meningitis may be the predominant feature.

Laboratory diagnosis

The organism may be cultured from the blood and CSF in the early days of the illness and from the urine thereafter but this requires long incubation and is not always successful. Inoculation of guinea-pigs may be helpful. Direct dark field microscopy of blood, CSF or urinary sediment is unrewarding. Serological investigation may be by complement fixation tests which will establish the presence of antibodies in the patient's serum to the genus generally. More detailed identification for epidemiological purposes depends on agglutination tests of considerable complexity.

Treatment

It is probably useful to treat leptospirosis in the first few days of illness with large doses of penicillin of 5–10 mega units. Treatment at later stages is certainly less likely to be effective.

Relapsing Fever

This disease, which is rare in Western Europe, is caused by spirochaetes of the genus borrelia. Two main species are involved: *Borrelia recurrentis* and *Borrelia duttoni*. Both are arthropod-borne from person to person by the louse and tick respectively. After an incubation period of a few days there is a sudden onset of high pyrexia, headache, and generalized pains. Nausea and vomiting are common and jaundice and conjunctivitis occur. The temperature chart may show the typical drop to subnormal levels after about a week when there is a period of relief from pain although the patient is collapsed, weak, and ill. This apparent recovery occurs because antibodies produced in response to the borrelia have cleared them from the blood. They do however survive in the tissues and subsequently emerge. They are antigenically variable and it requires a new antibody response to control them. Thus in a week or 10 days the temperature may rise again in many patients and the symptoms return although less severely. The situation repeats itself, although usually in a diminishing proportion of patients and with decreasing severity as the antibody response becomes increasingly effective. Louse borne relapsing fever is usually more severe than the tick borne type.

The organism is a short, motile, spiral spirochaete 6–10μ in length with loose waves of about 5–10 in number. It can be seen especially in louse borne infection in the peripheral blood using dark ground microscopy or Giemsa stain.

Treatment of established infection is by tetracycline or penicillin and a single dose may be effective, although the danger of a serious Jarisch-Herxheimer reaction should be anticipated (Chapter VII).

GENERALIZED RICKETTSIAL INFECTIONS

The rickettsiae are a group of very small Gram-negative cocco-bacilli about 0.3μ in diameter. They can be distinguished from viruses by their possession of both DNA and RNA but they cannot reproduce outside living cells. The diseases they cause in man are carried to him by insect vectors. The rickettsiae enter the body and after spreading in the blood stream infect the endothelial lining of the capillaries of the skin, CNS and heart. There they form small nodules packed with leucocytes and macrophages.

Louse Typhus (Epidemic or classical)

Infecting organism

Rickettsia prowazeki.

Vector

The body louse of man, *Pediculus corporis.*

Clinical features

This very serious disease is transferred to man by infected louse faeces contaminating scratches on the skin around its bite. There is an incubation period of 1-3 weeks followed by a period of 1 or 2 days of headache, nausea and vomiting, and generalized pains. A rise in temperature follows with intense headache and the development of drowsy stupor. A macular rash develops about the fifth day of illness, spreading over the trunk, thighs, and upper arms. The disease carries a very high mortality in older patients, usually from heart or renal failure. The disease was at one time common throughout the world and serious epidemics involved millions of people. With improved conditions and the use of insecticides it has been absent from Western Europe for several decades but is still endemic in parts of the 'Third World'.

Laboratory diagnosis

This depends on demonstration of the 'Weil–Felix Reaction' and more specifically by complement fixation tests for antibodies in the serum. The Weil–Felix reaction depends on the ability of the serum of the patient to agglutinate suspensions of three different strains of proteus, presumably due to some antigen shared by these strains and the rickettsiae. Different rickettsiae can be differentiated to some extent by varying reactions between their antibodies and the proteus strains.

Treatment

In the early stages of the infection there is a good response to tetracycline. Lice should be killed by widespread use of DDT or other insecticide. Typhus vaccine made from formalin-inactivated *Rickettsia prowazeki*, given in two doses subcutaneously, gives good protection. Most important in eradicating typhus is the improvement of living standards and hygiene.

Other Forms of Rickettsial Infection

There is a wide variety of other rickettsial diseases carried by various vectors and common in different parts of the world. Some of these are shown in Table X.2. In none of them is the illness so severe as typhus. In all of them the normal host is not man but a rodent. They respond well to treatment with tetracycline.

Table X.2

Disease	Normal host	Vector to man	Rickettsia
Murine typhus	Rat	Flea	*R. prowazeki var mooseri*
Scrub typhus	Rat	Mite	*R. tsutsugamushi*
Rocky Mountain Spotted Fever	Rodent	Tick	*R. rickettsia*
Tick Fever	Rodent	Tick	*R. australis*, *R. conori*
Rickettsial Pox	Mouse	Mite	*R. akari*

'Q' Fever (Query Fever)

The causative organism of this disease, *Coxiella burneti*, is not a true rickettsia, being smaller and proving more resistant to drying. It is enzootic in sheep, cows, goats and some other animals in many parts of the world. Spread to man is not by way of the ticks which carry it from animal to animal but by ingestion of the organism in milk or by inhalation of dust. The disease usually presents as an atypical pneumonia but the liver and spleen are also affected and may be enlarged. Rarely endocarditis may occur as a complication. Treatment is by tetracycline.

CHAPTER XI

Generalized Mycotic Infections

Systemic mycotic infections are severe and often fatal. They are relatively rare in Western Europe and those which occur, do so most often endogenously in patients with low resistance naturally or nosocomially or following prolonged antibiotic therapy. However, in other parts of the world exogenous infections may commonly occur due to a variety of fungal agents present in the environment.

CANDIDIASIS

This is usually an endogenous infection. Altered resistance or changed conditions within the body allow the overgrowth of saprophytic *Candida albicans* in a variety of sites giving rise to opportunistic infection. Infections of the bowel, vagina, mouth, and skin are discussed in the appropriate chapters. The infection can occur in any part of the body including the lungs, urinary tract, meninges, and pericardium. Diagnosis is by direct microscopy and by culture of tissues or body fluids on blood agar or Sabouraud's agar which may demonstrate the large Gram-positive budding yeast.

Systemic candidiasis is probably best treated by flucytosine in combination with amphotericin B. Local manifestations can be treated by topical nystatin or clotrimazole. A number of other species of candida including *Candida tropicalis* occasionally cause endogenous infection in man.

ASPERGILLOSIS

Infecting organism

The aspergilli are moulds which produce a mycelium with septate hyphae and characteristically reproduce by asexual conidia. A reproductive conidiophore bears finger-like cells called sterigmata on which are short chains of conidia. They can be found in man as part of the normal flora of the respiratory tract and mouth. In conditions favourable to them they can produce disease usually in the lung or in the ear.

Clinical features

Aspergillus fumigatus is most frequently seen in the lung, *Aspergillus niger* in the ear. Aspergilloma occurs, after damage to the lung by other agents, as a circumscribed mass of mycelium. There is no invasion of lung tissue and the lesion may be symptomless. Aspergillosis of the lung occurs in conditions of reduced resistance and immunosuppression and is associated with steroid therapy. There is a true infection with invasion of lung tissue. Aspergillus otitis externa follows bacterial infection of the outer ear. It can often be readily recognized on auroscopy when the typical black heads of the conidiophores of *Aspergillus niger* can be seen.

Laboratory diagnosis

The presence of an aspergillus in sputum is insufficient to allow diagnosis of infection. Repeated recognition and isolation should give rise to suspicion. Serum antibodies can be demonstrated by CIE and are a helpful indicator of infection.

Treatment

Generalized infections of the lung or other organs may require intravenous amphotericin B, possibly best combined with flucytosine. Aspergilloma does not respond well to antimycotics. Ear infections may be best treated by topical agents. When there has been spread to sinuses, surgical drainage should be carried out.

COCCIDIOIDOMYCOSIS

This infection is found in sunny, arid parts of the USA but it may be imported to other countries by returning travellers.

Infecting organism

Coccidioides immitis is a fungus normally found in dry soil. Here it forms a mycelium in the soil from which develop arthroconidia which release spores into the air and ensure its spread. This is its saprophytic cycle. If the spores are inhaled by man or some other animals a parasitic cycle may begin.

Clinical features

The majority of infections are asymptomatic but in those affected there is an incubation period of 1–3 weeks followed by development of cough, fever, chest pain, and malaise with sweating and rigors. Recovery is normally expected but occasionally the disease may become chronic especially in those with lowered resistance. Lung cavities may develop. Very rarely the disease may become disseminated with the meninges and the bones and joints often affected and a fatal outcome not uncommon.

Laboratory diagnosis

The sputum or any other material should be searched for typical fungi. The organism can be grown in the laboratory but it should be remembered that it is a dangerous laboratory pathogen.

Skin testing with coccidioides antigen is positive within 3 weeks and thereafter antibodies can be demonstrated in the serum by immuno-diffusion. The present of IgM indicates recent infection. A positive complement fixation test is an indicator of disseminated infection.

Treatment

Serious or disseminated cases can be treated with intravenous amphotericin B. Surgical removal of chronic lung cavities should be done.

CRYPTOCOCCOSIS

Infecting organism

Cryptococcus neoformans is a yeast-like fungus which is widespread in soil in much of the world. The organism is probably inhaled in dust or dried pigeon droppings. Most often the infection is not clinically apparent but in some patients, particularly those of low resistance, the lungs are affected, with cough and chest pain. Later the infection may spread especially to the central nervous system where it causes a wide variety of symptoms, meningitis, weakness, dizziness, behavioural abnormality, diplopia, and nerve palsies. Hydrocephalus may be a complication and CNS disease is often fatal.

Laboratory diagnosis

The organism may be seen in, and cultured from, the sputum or from the CSF. The CSF protein is raised with an increase in white cells, mainly lymphocytes. Antigens may be demonstrated in the CSF.

Treatment

Amphotericin B intravenously with flucytosine orally should be continued for 6–8 weeks.

BLASTOMYCOSIS

North American blastomycosis is due to a dimorphic fungus, *Blastomyces dermatitidis*, which exists in soil as a mould but which when grown on laboratory media at 37°C appears as a yeast. It is probably inhaled in dust and spreads from the lung to involve any organ of the body but especially the skin, liver, spleen, kidneys, and bones. Symptomatology varies with the sites infected. The organism can be seen as a yeast in pus or scrapings from skin lesions. The disease is fatal in about 50% of cases. Treatment is by intravenous amphotericin B.

HISTOPLASMOSIS

Infecting organism

This systemic mycosis is due to infection with *Histoplasma capsulatum*. This is a dimorphic fungus appearing as a mould in soil in many parts of the world. When grown at 37°C or in human tissue it is seen as a yeast.

Clinical features

The fungus is probably inhaled in dust and may cause infection of the lung of varying severity or an asymptomatic infection. Patients with lowered resistance are most affected and in them there is more probability of spread throughout the body, with the liver, spleen, meninges, and the mucous membranes of the mouth and throat involved. The disease may become chronic.

Laboratory diagnosis

The organism can be demonstrated in and cultured from sputum, or material from ulcers and biopsies but the diagnosis is often made serologically by complement fixation. Skin tests with 'histoplasmin' are helpful but may cause false positive serology.

Treatment

This is with amphotericin B intravenously.

MUCORMYCOSIS

The Mucoraceae exist in the soil and elsewhere in nature and are presumably inhaled and ingested frequently by man. In a few individuals with decreased resistance, and especially in diabetes and immuno-suppression, they may invade the blood vessels and spread through them as large non-septate hyphae with right-angle branches. The nose, sinuses, and the brain are often affected (rhinocerebral mucormycosis) but the lung and the gastro-intestinal tract may also be involved. Treatment is by controlling or relieving the predisposing condition, surgical drainage when indicated and amphotericin B intravenously.

CHAPTER XII

Generalized Viral Infections

CHILDHOOD FEVERS

Measles

This very common disease of childhood is not usually a serious infection in the advanced urban societies. It is very infectious and by the end of childhood there is almost universal immunity to it. It does occur as a much more serious infection of adults and children in isolated communities without immunity and in areas where malnutrition and other diseases have lowered resistance.

Infecting organism

The measles virus is a paramyxovirus, infectious only to man and some primates.

Clinical features

Infection is by inhalation of droplets and is followed by an incubation period of 10–14 days. There is characteristically a prodromal respiratory illness during this period, with catarrh and conjunctivitis, then followed by the onset of fever and the development of the typical maculo-papular rash which persists for 4–5 days. During both the prodromal and overt phases there is viraemia. Clinical diagnosis depends on the rash and the observation of Koplik's spots which appear towards the end of the prodromal phase on the buccal mucosa as raised grey specks surrounded by erythema.

Laboratory diagnosis

This is rarely necessary as the clinical picture is clear, but during the prodromal phase typical giant cells may be seen in the sputum and nasal secretions. The virus itself may be isolated in tissue culture in the late prodromal and early stages of the rash from washings of the throat and nose. Serological diagnosis is more commonly used and antibodies can be demonstrated by complement fixation from a few days after the appearance of the rash.

Complications

The importance of measles in developed countries lies in the incidence of complications. Pneumonia and otitis media are more likely in the very young. Encephalomyelitis is a complication in about one case in one thousand, and has a mortality of 20%; and those who survive may show evidence of neurological damage.

Sub-acute sclerosing pan-encephalitis (SSPE) occurs rarely in those who have suffered from measles many years before, probably as the result of reactivation of the virus. The patients have a high titre of measles antibodies in their serum and the virus has been isolated from the brain of some fatal cases.

Immunization

The incidence of complications justifies a vaccination programme using attenuated live virus. Lasting immunity appears to be obtained with just one subcutaneous injection given at between 1 and 2 years. Passive immunity can be achieved by giving pooled human gamma globulin to protect measles contacts who are immunosuppressed or are in some way at special risk. In some advanced countries the disease has been wellnigh eradicated by immunization programmes.

Treatment

There is no treatment other than general nursing care. Secondary infections should be treated if necessary.

Rubella

This very common infection of childhood is usually so mild that it may pass undiagnosed. It is only moderately infectious and about 12–15% of people do not develop immunity during childhood. The importance of rubella lies in the damage it can cause to the foetus when the disease is contracted by the mother in early pregnancy.

Infecting organism

The virus is not unequivocally related to any group and is regarded as a rubivirus, a separate genus of the Togaviridae family.

Clinical features

The infection is spread by droplet inhalation and the incubation period is usually 18–20 days. In children the first sign is generally the appearance of a maculo-papular rash with possible cervical adenitis, catarrh and conjunctivitis. There is viraemia before the rash and until it fades in 4–5 days, and the patient is infectious before and after the appearance of the rash. Sub-clinical cases are also infectious.

Laboratory diagnosis

Because the consequences of rubella in pregnancy are so serious, laboratory tests must be used to give definitive diagnosis. The virus can be isolated from throat swabs and other body fluids but the important diagnostic test is the demonstration of a rising titre of antibodies and especially the demonstration of the presence of IgM indicating an acute infection. The importance of serological testing is to determine whether a women in the first months of pregnancy who is exposed to infection has already a protective titre of antibodies from previous natural infection or immunization, or whether she has no immunity and possibly has an acute infection.

Complications

Complications of rubella are rare. Arthritis may occur in a few adult cases and very rarely encephalitis.

Congenital rubella

The rubella virus passes the placenta and if the infection is contracted by the mother early in pregnancy there is a very considerable likelihood that the foetus will be damaged. The risk and severity of damage decreases with the age of the foetus and is minimal after 4 months. Damage includes spontaneous abortion, cataract, deafness, and congenital heart disease. Multiple defects occur in a single child especially in infection of very young foetuses. Babies born with congenital rubella are very infectious.

Immunization

There has been a prolonged campaign to immunize actively pre-pubertal schoolgirls. In addition there has been widespread testing of women in pregnancy for the presence of antibodies, followed by immediately post-partum immunization of those not immune. As a result the incidence of congenital rubella has fallen dramatically but the situation can only be maintained by continued immunization. A live attenuated vaccine is used in a single dose subcutaneously. It must not be given to a woman in pregnancy or to any woman likely to become pregnant within 2 months.

Treatment

There is no specific treatment.

Mumps

This commonly presents as a childhood infection involving the salivary glands but it may be more serious in the adult.

Infecting organism

The virus of mumps is a spherical paramyxovirus.

Clinical features

The virus is spread by droplet inhalation and the incubation period is 16–20 days. Prodromal symptoms are brief, with malaise and headache, and are rapidly followed by inflammation and enlargement of the parotid glands with difficulty in speaking and chewing. The condition may often be unilateral but is more commonly bilateral. The submandibular and submaxillary glands are occasionally involved. The swelling subsides in a week.

In post-pubertal patients it causes epididymo-orchitis in a quarter of males and oöphoritis in a very few women. Rarely, reduced fertility may follow these conditions.

Some degree of meningism occurs in a few cases and meningitis is a rare complication. Mumps is such a common infection however that this small proportion represents the most common cause of viral meningitis.

Laboratory diagnosis

This is not often necessary as the clinical diagnosis is usually obvious. A rising titre of antibodies can be demonstrated by complement fixation. The organism elaborates two main antigens. A soluble 'S' antigen from the viral nucleus predominates in the acute phase while in old infections only the 'V' surface antigen may be found. Testing for antibodies to these separate antigens by complement fixation can differentiate the phases of the disease. The CSF in mumps often shows increased white cells mainly lymphocytes.

Treatment

There is no specific treatment. *live attenuated.*

Varicella and Herpes Zoster

Varicella is a mild febrile contagious disease of children in which the patient is invaded for the first time by the varicella-zoster virus. Subsequently as an adult the virus may be reactivated in a nerve root ganglion as herpes zoster.

Infecting organism

The virus is of the herpes group and is an icosahedron formed by capsomeres and surrounded by a loose outer envelope.

Clinical features

(a) Varicella

The disease usually of children is transmitted from patients with either varicella or herpes-zoster by inhalation of droplets from the mouth lesions or particles from the skin lesions. There is an incubation period of about 15 days followed by the appearance of the vesicular rash which affects first the trunk and then the arms, legs, and face with vesicles also in the mouth and throat. Detailed interest in the rash in varicella is now of less importance as the differential diagnosis of smallpox is no longer vital.

(b) Herpes Zoster

This occurs in the adult as a reactivation of the virus usually in a dorsal nerve root or sometimes in a cranial nerve. There is a vesicular eruption of the skin over the area of distribution of the sensory nerve or nerves affected.

Laboratory diagnosis

The organism can be seen in vesicle fluid and antibodies demonstrated in the serum. This has lost importance since the disappearance of smallpox and the need for differential diagnosis.

Complications

Post varicella encephalitis occasionally occurs and adults often suffer pneumonic infection during the disease. The virus passed the placenta and infants can be born suffering from neonatal varicella.

Treatment

There is no specific therapy in simple varicella except to avoid secondary infection. The pain and the duration of the rash in zoster can be relieved with idoxuridine applied to the affected area.

HEPATITIS

Viral hepatitis has been divided into two quite separate conditions, hepatitis A and hepatitis B. Recently further forms of viral hepatitis have been described and are at the moment grouped as 'Non A, non B' hepatitis.

Hepatitis A (Infectious hepatitis)

This is usually a relatively mild infection of children and young people which may often be sub-clinical but which may give rise to low pyrexia with nausea and vomiting and jaundice. It is widespread throughout the world and has a low mortality of about one in a thousand.

Infecting organism

This is not clearly defined but particles of 27 nm have been demonstrated in the faeces of hepatitis patients by electron microscopy and have been specifically aggregated by serum from convalescent cases.

Clinical features

The disease is spread from person to person by the faecal–oral route, usually occurring as single sporadic cases except in closed communities where outbreaks may occur. Occasionally it may occur as a food or water-borne epidemic. The incubation period is 15–40 days following which there is a pre-icteric phase of the disease with nausea, anorexia, headache, vomiting, and low grade pyrexia. Within a few days this is succeeded by the icteric phase with frank jaundice accompanied by dark urine and pale stools and pruritis. Occasionally the disease may be severe with fulminant hepatic failure and sometimes death. The virus is present in the faeces during the incubation period and pre-icteric phase but is less easily found thereafter.

Laboratory diagnosis

Biochemistry of the serum is valuable to establish that there is acute hepatitis. The demonstration of the virus in the stools and its specific aggregation is a difficult procedure. Antibodies to the virus appear in the serum early in the disease and are best demonstrated by radioimmune assay. A fourfold rise in titre between an acute and convalescent serum is necessary for diagnosis, as many people have some antibody to hepatitis A virus. Demonstration of IgM antibody in a single sample can be diagnostic. The absence of serological evidence of hepatitis B is in itself a helpful diagnostic pointer.

Treatment

There is no specific treatment. Prophylactic passive immunization of contacts or those at special risk can be achieved by giving normal human immunoglobulin as soon as possible after exposure. Travellers to areas where hepatitis A is common may be offered immunoglobulin and one injection will give some protection for several months.

Hepatitis B (Serum Hepatitis)

This is a widespread infection which affects a significant proportion of people in most communities especially in less developed countries. It is very often a sub-clinical infection but may give rise to a serious and prolonged illness. It arises as a natural infection but is also of great concern because of its occurrence following transfer by injection or transfusion where infected needles, instruments, blood or blood products carry the organism to the patient. There is a high incidence therefore among those receiving multiple transfusions, patients in renal dialysis units, drug addicts, and those being tattooed. Indeed all patients receiving injections and all nursing, medical, and dental staff are also theoretically at risk. Danger arises not only from cases of hepatitis B but also from carriers who may be a source of infection to others. Carriers continue after frank or sub-clinical infection for periods of months or years to maintain active infectious virus in blood and other secretions. They must be excluded by laboratory screening from blood donation or from renal dialysis units and specimens from them must be handled with care (Chapter XIV).

Infecting organism

The hepatitis B virus can be taken to be a particle 42 nm in diameter, the Dane particle, which together with smaller fragments is found in serum from hepatitis patients.

Clinical features

Hepatitis B is classically transferred by injection or transfusion or may be acquired naturally by passage in saliva, faecal–orally, or during sexual intercourse or in any natural contact with infected blood, urine or other body fluids. It is a sporadic infection and epidemics do not occur. The incubation period is relatively long, being 2–5 months. There is an insidious onset, with fever and rash preceding an icteric phase. There have been a few instances of serious infections with significant mortality occurring in numbers of patients and staff in hospital units, and there seems no doubt that a serious situation can develop especially in renal dialysis and transplant units. This has resulted in very considerable emphasis on hepatitis B as a nosocomial disease and an occupational hazard.

Laboratory diagnosis

In the course of infection a number of antigens can be recognized. Surface antigen HB_sAg, core antigen HB_cAg and another antigen HB_eAg, whose site of origin is less clear, can be demonstrated. Surface antigen, once called Australia Antigen, appears in the serum several weeks before the clinical symptoms and often for many weeks to follow. The titres of the antigens rise usually until the onset of jaundice and fall thereafter. The antibodies to the antigens can be recognized in the convalescent phase.

Carriers maintain HB_SAg in their serum while HB_CAg which also persists can be suddenly replaced by Anti HB_C and the demonstration of Anti $HB_C IgM$ can be indicative of a carrier state. Carriers of HB_eAg are considered to be particularly infectious and can transmit hepatitis apparently by very small infecting doses.

Treatment

There is no specific treatment. In prophylaxis normal human immuno-globulin is not effective but specific anti-hepatitis B globulin can be used where an obvious risk has been run or injury sustained. A vaccine to allow active immunization against hepatitis B has recently been developed.

'Non A, Non B' Hepatitis

This form of hepatitis is caused by a virus other than A or B, but it is usually transmitted in the same way as hepatitis B and is associated with blood and blood products. Human immunoglobulin can be used to give prophylactic protection.

SMALLPOX

It appears increasingly probable as the years pass without report of a case of naturally acquired smallpox, that this great scourge of mankind has been eradicated from the world. There is still the chance of accidental laboratory infection and it is possible also that in the future some variation of monkeypox or similar infection may adapt itself successfully to man.

The factors which made the eradication of smallpox possible are worth considering. It has no natural animal reservoir, so that measures against it could be concentrated entirely on human cases. An attack of smallpox conferred good and lasting immunity. Active artificial immunization by attenuated vaccine was effective and safe and although the immunity did not last well at a high level it was easily boosted by repeat vaccinations. Together with a policy of isolation of known cases, vaccination of contacts and of susceptible populations gradually confined the disease to smaller remote areas and the last reported case occurred in the Horn of Africa in 1978. None has been reported since and it would seem that the apparently impossible dream of removing a major infectious disease completely from the world is indeed a reality.

THE VIRAL HAEMORRHAGIC FEVERS

Lassa, Marburg and Ebola fever are often grouped together although caused by different agents. They occur in Africa endemically but they are all fortunately extremely rare elsewhere. Travellers incubating these fevers may however arrive in other areas.

Lassa Fever

Infecting organism

Named after the Nigerian town in which it was first recognized, Lassa fever is caused by an arenavirus.

Clinical features

The disease seems to occur quite frequently in West Africa, where in some areas considerable numbers of the population show serological evidence of past infection. It occurs naturally in a small rodent, *Mastomys natalensis*, whence it spreads to humans possibly by way of infected urine. Spread from person to person does seem to occur and it is this aspect of the disease which has caused great reaction and activity among those who must care for cases in this country.

The incubation period is variable from a few days to 2 weeks, following which a serious fever develops with malaise, cough, sore throat, headache, vomiting, abdominal pain, and diarrhoea. There is a considerable mortality and in view of the danger to medical attendants known cases are nursed strictly in isolators. Obviously in Africa the disease must follow a less serious course among the people native to the area at least on some occasions.

Laboratory diagnosis

Laboratory specimens should only be examined in special Category A Pathogen Laboratories.

Treatment

The only treatment is passive immunization using convalescent human serum.

Marburg Fever and Ebola Fever

Infecting organisms

Both viruses are RNA-containing and may be long branching structures. They are distinguishable serologically.

Clinical features

The number of epidemics studied is limited. Imported African vervet monkeys have transmitted Marburg fever to hospital workers in Europe before succumbing themselves. The source of the disease which infected the monkeys is not known. Ebola virus has caused outbreaks in central Africa, several hundred people being affected with a mortality of more than 50%. The diseases are severe haemorrhagic fevers with onset after a few days incubation of headache, fever, malaise, vomiting, diarrhoea and muscle pains. The rash follows and is haemorrhagic. There is marked intravascular coagulation which leads to death.

Laboratory diagnosis

This should only be attempted in Category A Pathogen Laboratories.

Treatment

Only convalescent serum is at present available to give some protection. Strict isolation of cases must be practised.

YELLOW FEVER

A group of toga viruses, arthropod borne, cause a wide variety of encephalitis and haemorrhagic fevers throughout the old and new world. Vectors include mosquitoes, ticks and sandflies. Yellow fever is widespread in tropical Africa and Central and South America. It is enzootic in various monkeys and is passed to man by the bite of an infected *Aëdes aëgypti* or certain other mosquitoes.

Infecting organism

The toga viruses are RNA-containing icosahedral particles.

Clinical features

There is sudden onset with fever, headache, abdominal pain, vomiting and myalgia. Jaundice develops and in serious and fatal cases haemorrhage with blood in the stools and 'coffee ground' vomit.

Laboratory diagnosis

The virus can be isolated by inoculation of blood or tissue into suckling mice. Serology by demonstrating haemagglutination inhibition (HI) antibodies or complement fixation can be useful.

Treatment

There is no specific treatment. Immunization using a live attenuated vaccine is very effective and following one dose there is immunity for up to 10 years. It is absolutely vital that anyone proceeding to or passing through a yellow fever area be vaccinated.

CHAPTER XIII

Generalized Protozoal Infections

MALARIA

Malaria is one of the most serious and widespread infections of man, affecting millions of people throughout Africa, Central and South America, and the Middle and Far East. The infecting protozoan is inoculated into man by a female *Anopheles* mosquito feeding on his blood.

Infecting organism

Human malaria is caused by a number of species of *Plasmodium* : *vivax*, *ovale*, *malariae* or *falciparum*. Infection may occur with more than one of these species and occasionally other species are involved. The life cycle of the plasmodia is basically similar for all species (Fig. XIII.1).

1) Pre-erythrocytic cycle

In the course of sucking human blood the Anopheles mosquito inoculates man with sporozoites in its saliva. These enter parenchymatous cells in the liver and divide to form schizonts which are filled with large numbers of merozoites. The schizont ruptures releasing macromerozoites to invade further liver cells, and micromerozoites to invade the blood stream and its red cells. This pre-erythrocytic phase occupies about 1 week.

2) Exo-erythrocytic cycle

The macromerozoites enter further parenchymatous liver cells and repeat the process described above at intervals of a few days and persist in the liver thereafter. This occurs with *P. malariae*, *vivax*, and *ovale* but *P. falciparum* does not have a persisting exo-erythrocytic cycle after the initial pre-erythrocytic phase.

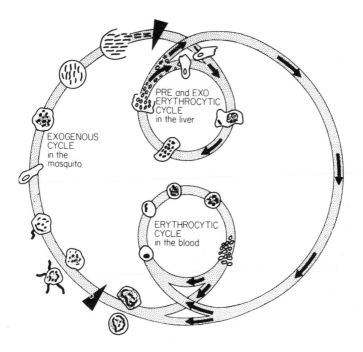

Figure XIII.1   Life cycle of malaria parasite

3) Erythrocytic cycle

Micromerozoites enter red cells in the circulating blood and develop into trophozoites which appear as ring forms and mature to form schizonts consisting of daughter merozoites. The cell ruptures, releasing these into the blood where they invade other red cells and repeat the cycle. This occurs as a 48 hour cycle in *P. vivax, ovale,* and *falciparum* and a 72 hour cycle in *P. malariae.* Some of the merozoites develop within the red cells into male microgametocytes and some into female macrogametocytes. These sexual forms are large round structures filling the host red cell or in the case of *P. falciparum* distorting it into a long oval shape. They do not reproduce in the human host but form the mechanism of infection of the blood-sucking Anopheles mosquito and the life cycle within its body.

4) Exogenous cycle

After entering the stomach of the mosquito the gametocytes break out of the erythrocytes and develop to form gametes. In the case of the male gametocyte, slender flagella appear on its surface and break free into the stomach as microgametes. There they move to the female gamete and fertilize it to form a zygote. This becomes oval in shape and penetrates the stomach lining as an ookinete, where it forms as an oocyst packed with slender sporozoites which rupture from it into the body cavity of the mosquito and spread throughout its body including the salivary glands. The infected saliva is inoculated into man when the mosquito next sucks blood.

Clinical features

Although malaria is endemic only in those parts of the world sufficiently warm to permit the survival of the *Anopheles* mosquito, the disease is seen frequently in Europe and North America in returning travellers. The diagnosis must always be considered as the infection can be serious and even fatal. *P. malariae* is found world wide. *P. vivax* predominates in the Indian sub-continent and Central America, *P. falciparum* in Africa, where *P. ovale* also occurs, and both *vivax* and *falciparum* are found in the Far East and South America.

Although there are considerable differences in the symptoms, severity, and periodicity in malaria due to the different species of plasmodia there is a basic similarity. Following inoculation by the mosquito there is an incubation period of about 12–15 days. This may be much longer especially if the number of sporozoites injected is small or if the patient has some prophylactic protection. Following this there is malaise, then chills and rigors, a high pyrexia and then profuse sweating and a drop in the temperature. This cycle is then repeated at intervals which may be daily (quotidian) at first or irregular but may settle to a characteristic periodicity thereafter, varying with the species of plasmodium involved. Falciparum malaria can frequently be fatal in primary infection with jaundice, renal failure, circulatory collapse or cerebral involvement with delirium and coma. Early anti-malarial treatment is essential or death may ensue. All forms of malaria may be accompanied by splenomegaly, hepatomegaly and some degree of anaemia. The spleen may sometimes be easily ruptured due to its sudden enlargement.

Following a period of a few weeks the untreated infection resolves but relapses are very common and may occur over many years in some types of malaria.

Laboratory diagnosis

The malarial parasites should be demonstrated in the peripheral blood by repeated examination if necessary. Thick blood films are used to detect the parasites. It may be helpful to lyse the blood cells with distilled water or saponin and stain with Giemsa. Thin blood films are required to speciate the parasites using Giemsa or Leishman's stain (Fig. I,8). Speciation requires experience and depends on a number of characteristics of the parasite and the host red cell.

It may be of value to carry out sternal puncture if the peripheral blood is negative, as the parasite is generally more numerous in the bone marrow. Serological tests to demonstrate malarial antibodies are of little diagnostic value. They become positive about a week after symptoms appear but persist for years.

Treatment

Malaria due to *P. vivax, malariae*, and *ovale* is best treated using chloroquine, a 4-aminoquinoline. This is effective against the erythrocytic schizonts and gametocytes but leaves the exo-erythrocytic cycle intact, which may have some benefit in maintaining immunity in those liable to repeated exposure. In others if it is desirable to try to eradicate the exo-erythrocytic parasites an 8-aminoquinoline such as primaquine can be used immediately after the chloroquine regime is complete. It is given orally for 14 days.

Malaria due to *P. falciparum* can also be treated by chloroquine. *P. falciparum* does not have an exo-erythrocytic cycle. Unfortunately many strains of falciparum are now resistant to chloroquine especially in certain countries of South East Asia and in these cases a course of quinine can be given orally, every 8 hours for 2 days followed after that regimen by a single oral dose of pyrimethamine and sulphadoxine. These are combined in appropriate proportions in 'Fansidar' a commercial preparation.

Prophylaxis

It is absolutely essential that any traveller entering a malarial area, however briefly, should be protected by chemoprophylactics. A number of drugs are available and those commonly advised are chloroquine which is given weekly or proguanil given daily.

Chloroquine-resistant *P. falciparum* has emerged in many countries and there it is necessary to use weekly pyrimethine-sulphadoxine. The situation is not static and up to date local advice on prophylaxis must be sought. It is vital that prophylaxis be started before entering a malarial area and continued for 4 weeks after leaving it.

Control

The control of malaria involves several lines of attack. The *Anopheles* mosquito should be destroyed directly by the use of insecticides. Its potential breeding grounds in ponds, ditches and all shaded stagnant surface water should be reduced by drainage, good hygiene and by treating the water surface with oil or introducing fish which eat the mosquito larvae. The mosquito should be prevented from biting by mosquito nets, long trousers and sleeves. Homes should be mosquito proof. Chemoprophylaxis and chemotherapy act by preventing the mosquito from becoming infected by the gametocytes. An acceptable vaccine against malaria is not yet available.

AFRICAN TRYPANOSOMIASIS

This disease, commonly known as sleeping sickness, affects an enormous part of West, Central, and East Africa, depopulating entire areas and rendering them uninhabitable.

Infecting organism

Two haemoflagellates (Fig. XIII,2), distinguishable from each other only by their effect on man and by the vector which carries them to him,

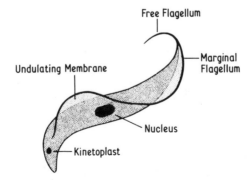

Figure XIII.2 *Trypanosoma brucei gambiense*

are responsible for sleeping sickness. *Trypanosoma brucei gambiense* is carried to man by riverine tsetse flies. It causes disease in West and Central Africa and as far east as Uganda and Southern Sudan. It is a human parasite and is spread by the fly from man to man.

Trypanosoma brucei rhodesiense is naturally a parasite of the bush buck and is adapted to man. It is normally carried by another tsetse fly from the buck to man, but it can pass via the fly from man to man in epidemic conditions.

The trypanosomes appear in the blood as small, pointed, slender organisms with a free flagellum at the anterior end continuing as a marginal flagellum on the edge of an undulating membrane for the greater part of the body length to a kinetoplast at the posterior end. The nucleus is central.

Clinical features

Following the bite of the tsetse fly and the inoculation of the trypanosome, there is a local tissue reaction, the primary chancre. The organisms then enter the lymph and blood giving rise to fever, weakness, anaemia and lymphadenitis. This typically appears in the posterior trangle of the neck. This period lasts for a few months in rhodesiense infections and for a few years in gambiense infections before the CNS is invaded and cerebral trypanosomiasis, sleeping sickness, is established. This is a chronic meningo-encephalomyelitis giving rise to progressive mental deterioration. The patient has a slow shuffling gait, mask-like expression, tremors and indistinct speech. He falls asleep by day, loses interest in all activity including eating and dies in coma or often of intercurrent infection.

Laboratory diagnosis

Thick blood films stained by Giemsa should be examined for the organisms and blood containing anticoagulant can be concentrated by centrifugation. The protozoan can be seen in aspirate from lymph glands and in the centrifuged deposit from the CSF. The ESR and the serum IgM rise to very high levels and can be helpful diagnostic points.

Treatment

Treatment with arsenicals can be very effective. Prophylaxis is not very satisfactory but drugs can give some protection against gambiense infection.

Control

Control of the vector and avoidance of its bite can be very difficult. Major movement of population from tsetse fly infested areas to clear areas has been effective but has obvious difficulties and limitations. Large areas of Africa are still unusuable because of this infection.

SOUTH AMERICAN TRYPANOSOMIASIS (CHAGA'S DISEASE)

The disease occurs widely throughout much of South America. The causative protozoan is *Trypanosoma cruzi* and the vector is one of a variety of reduviid bugs. The organism enters the body from the bug faeces, probably scratched into its bite. The disease follows a local reaction period and spreads through the body. The spleen and liver are enlarged and there are multiple wide-spread granulomata. The CNS is not invaded but the autonomic system is affected. Death follows years later from heart failure and general debility. Diagnosis is by demonstration of the organism in the blood. There is no effective treatment.

LEISHMANIASIS

Visceral Leishmaniasis (Kala-azar)

This disease is found widely spread in Central and North Africa, the Middle and Far East, and some parts of South America. It is due to infection by a parasite, *Leishmania donovani*, which is introduced to man by the bite of an infected sandfly (*Phlebotomus*).

Infecting organism

In the sandfly the organism appears in a long, slender form, flagellated and motile. When this organism is inoculated by the sandfly into man or animals it develops as a small, oval form with a large nucleus and a rod-shaped kinetoplast and is seen intracellularly in macrophages and reticulo-endothelial cells (Fig. XIII,3). The animal reservoirs vary in different parts of the world and include dogs, jackals, rodents, and man himself.

Clinical features

After the bite of an infected sandfly there is a long incubation period of

2–4 months, although this may vary considerably. This is followed by the onset of fever, often showing twice daily peaks at first and over a few weeks developing an undulating pattern. The spleen rapidly enlarges and the femoral and inguinal glands are enlarged and there is dark pigmentation of the skin in many cases. The condition may continue for months with enlargement of the liver at this stage. The blood shows anaemia, leucopenia, and thrombocytopenia, and haemorrhage and purpura are seen. Patients are very liable to intercurrent infections.

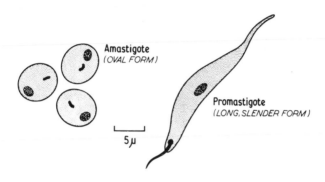

Figure XIII.3   *Leishmania donovani*

Laboratory diagnosis

The organism can be seen in blood, aspirated lymph nodes, bone marrow or spleen as the small round 'Leishman–Donovan Bodies' and can be cultured on special media where it assumes its slender form. Serological tests for antibodies can be helpful.

Treatment

Sodium stibogluconate, an organic antimony compound, for 4 weeks is effective except where resistance has developed, when pentamidine may be used.

Control

Attempts should be made to destroy sandflies with insecticides and to control the local host animal where this is possible.

Cutaneous leishmaniasis

Other leishmania not morphologically distinguishable from *Leishmania donovani* cause cutaneous and muco-cutaneous infections in Africa, Asia, and South and Central America. They are carried by sandflies.

TOXOPLASMOSIS

The disease is of world-wide distribution and is due to infection by a protozoan, *Toxoplasma gondii*. Man acts as an intermediate host for the organism and is generally not very susceptible to it. Infection can take place at any age and about 40% of adults show serological evidence of antibody production.

Infecting organism

Toxoplasma gondii is a protozoan related to the plasmodium of malaria. It is found in a wide variety of mammals, of which the cat is most important as a factor in human toxoplasmosis. The cat acts as a definitive host and the organism reproduces asexually in the mucosa of its small bowel. Sexual reproduction takes place also with the production of gametocytes, fertilization and production of a zygote which develops to an oöcyst. These cysts are discharged in the cat faeces for about 10 days after infection and infect man, who may inhale or ingest the cysts or they may enter abrasions on his skin. Children playing in the apparent safety of suburban gardens can be at considerable risk. The organism may also be ingested in uncooked meat, and abattoir workers may be infected through abrasions. The organism enters the lymphocytes and reticulo-endothelial cells and can be seen within cells and free in the blood as a boat-shaped trophozoite (Fig. XIII,4). Large cystic forms may also be seen in chronic toxoplasmosis.

Clinical features

Toxoplasma infection is normally asymptomatic but may cause fever, lymphadenopathy and sore throat. Chronic toxoplasmosis may follow and affect the eye, causing chorio-retinitis. The disease may occasionally be severe and result in spread to the CNS. Immunosuppressed patients are at greatest risk.

The major hazard to man lies in congenital toxoplasmosis. This occurs when a non-immune mother is infected in pregnancy, normally

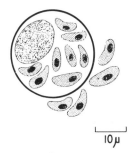

Intra and extra-cellular
Trophozoites

10 μ

Figure XIII.4   *Toxoplasma gondii*

asymptomatically. The protozoan passes the placenta and affects the
unborn child, being especially damaging in the first trimester. Abortion,
still-birth or a live but affected child may result with chrorioretinitis,
hydrocephalus, and other brain damage most commonly present.

Laboratory diagnosis

The organism can be seen in lymph node biopsies and may be cultivated
in mice from aspirates but diagnosis is usually serological. The classical
Dye Test depends on the ability of serum antibodies to prevent the
normal uptake of methylene blue by live toxoplasmas, and a high or
rising titre can be diagnostic. Complement fixation and the demonstration
of significant levels of specific IgM by fluorescence techniques are
indicative of recent infection.

Treatment

Acute infections of a serious nature can be treated using pyrimethamine
together with sulphonamides and folinic acid for 1–2 months. The
inapparent infection in pregnancy may well mean that there is no
opportunity for treatment. If an infection is proven it may be considered
that abortion of the foetus should be carried out. Spiramycin may be
used in pregnancy as a less hazardous alternative to pyrimethamine. The
screening of women in pregnancy for immunity to toxoplasmosis and for
evidence of infection during pregnancy is practised in some countries.
Awareness of being at special risk might be of value to the mother.

CHAPTER XIV

Hospital Infection

INTRODUCTION

The term 'Hospital Infection' in its widest sense embraces any infection which is acquired by a person while in hospital whether as patient, staff or visitor. It is, however, used in a more specific way to describe particular infections which occur in patients during their stay in hospital especially infections of wounds and burns and of their respiratory and urinary tracts. Intestinal infection when it arises and spreads in the hospital community must also be included.

Hospital infection has certain important characteristics in that the victims of it are relatively more susceptible and have less resistance than the normal population. They often are old or very young, they have a variety of debilitating conditions, and they may be receiving therapy such as steroids, cytotoxic drugs or irradiation which suppresses their immune response. Locally their tissues may have been damaged and exposed by accident or in operation. They may suffer urinary stasis or blockage or be unable to cough and have poor respiratory cilial function. The effect of modern anaesthetics and a major abdominal operation on the ability to clear the respiratory tract and to pass urine can be very considerable.

The conditions in hospital of close contact and intimate care give every opportunity for the spread of organism between patients themselves and between patients and staff. Invasion of the susceptible tissue of the patient is all too easy.

The organisms in the environment are themselves not entirely unaffected by the unusual factors applying in the hospital environment. Selective forces tend over years to favour invasive and virulent organisms and the particular favouring of organisms resistant to the antibiotics used in the hospital has meant the selection of species not usually associated with infection and sepsis outside hospital. Within species there is selection of resistant variants to the point at which they now form almost the entire hospital flora.

All these factors, the highly susceptible host, the simple pathways of spread and the selected hospital organisms together mean that hospital infection is a unique problem. Unlike for example an epidemic of measles which waxes, wanes and disappears or a sporadic infection such as tetanus which may affect one unfortunate individual, hospital infection is an endless continuous situation occurring in an enclosed environment. Any action taken in that environment affects the whole system, an antibiotic given to a patient does not just affect that patient for good or ill, it also contributes to the concentration of the antibiotic in the environment as a whole and to the development of resistance in the whole flora of the hospital. The introduction of an infected patient potentially introduces his organisms to all, unless he is successfully isolated. It is vital therefore that the nature, causes, sources, and spread of hospital infection be understood and that the preventive measures necessary to hold it in check are clearly formulated and followed by all.

WOUND INFECTIONS

While it is difficult to compare the statistical evidence of wound infection between one hospital and another or even between one ward and another, the average general hospital with normal standards can be expected to suffer about a 6% overall post-operative wound infection rate. The rate for clean elective surgery may be about 2% while contaminated injuries and surgery on the urinary tract and the lower bowel for example can be expected to yield a higher rate. Hospitals with poor standards can be much worse. The greater suffering of the individual patient whose wound is infected, the prolonged stay in hospital with its social and economic disruption, the cost to the community in extra care and lost production add up to a very significant problem indeed.

It is necessary to look first at what organisms are involved together with their origin in the patient, in the theatre and in the ward.

Infecting Organisms

Streptococcus pyogenes

Historically wound infection with the group A, β-haemolytic streptococci was the greatest scourge of surgery and obstetrics and resulted in such mortality as to induce patients to regard hospital admission for surgery as a death sentence. Improved hygiene, aseptic technique and then the introduction of penicillin and the failure of the streptococcus to adapt to resist it, has so reduced the incidence and severity of streptococcal infection that there is real danger of its being discounted. It can still be a serious hospital infection problem in neonates, post-natal infections and particularly infection of burns.

Staphylococcus aureus

The coagulase positive staphylococcus is now a major cause of hospital wound infection. Unlike the streptococcus it has adapted well to resist many antibiotics. The selection of strains producing a β-lactamase (penicillinase) able to destroy penicillin has meant that in hospital this antibiotic is useless against staphylococcal infection. However, staphylococcal wound infection, while serious, does not produce the morbidity or mortality associated once with streptococcal infection. The major difficulty in its control arises from its universal presence in the hospital environment, where it may be found on the skin and in the noses of patients and staff and in the dust on floors, bedclothes, furniture, and apparatus.

Gram-negative bacilli

These organisms are now the cause of the majority of wound sepsis in hospital. This is due partly to the natural antibiotic resistance of the organisms as compared with Gram-positive cocci, to their ability to become resistant to those antibiotics which are at first effective and to the large proportion of surgical wounds which involve the bowel and the urinary tract or the skin areas near them, where the Gram-negative organisims of the bowel abound. Coliforms including *Escherichia coli* itself, *Proteus* spp. klebsiellas and pseudomonads are those most often involved. The pseudomonads are almost exclusively hospital organisms not found in sepsis occurring outside. They are naturally and by adaptation extremely resistant and treatment of infection is very difficult. They often succeed finally other less resistant organisms to cause a terminal infection.

Anaerobes

Anaerobic infections may be due to *Clostridium perfringens* or *Clostridium tetani*, or other members of the clostridium group, to *Bacteroides* spp. or anaerobic streptocci. Except in rare circumstances these infections differ from other hospital wound infections in that they are sporadic single cases and there is no spread from patient to patient.

Other organisms

In suitable circumstances any pathogenic organism may infect a wound. In situations of reduced resistance other organisms not normally regarded as pathogenic may also do so and this is then referred to as an opportunistic infection. It should be remembered that an organism carried harmlessly in one site may be a pathogen in another. *Escherichia coli* in an adult bowel may be harmless but may be pathogenic in the urinary tract. A simple staphylococcus of the skin or a commensal viridans streptococcus of the respiratory tract may be a serious pathogen if it colonizes a damaged heart valve.

URINARY TRACT INFECTIONS

These are considered in general in Chapter VI. They do, however, form a significant proportion of hospital acquired infections, usually following surgical interference on the urinary tract and even simple urethral catheterization. The combination of the introduction of micro-organisms and the stasis of urinary flow which often occurs during or following surgery gives ideal circumstances for the development of infection.

RESPIRATORY TRACT INFECTIONS

These are discussed in Chapter IV. Additional hazards leading to respiratory infections in hospital are: anaesthesia, which suppresses coughing and the free movement of the cilia lining the tract and removing dust and mucus and micro-organisms; the natural fear of coughing which afflicts a patient with an abdominal wound; and the presence of hospital organisms which may colonize the patient. Infection of the trachea and the lungs in patients on assisted respiration is a difficult problem, and *Pseudomonas aeruginosa* infection is particularly hard to avoid.

INTESTINAL INFECTIONS

These are considered in Chapter VIII. They may occur in hospital and outbreaks due to salmonellae, shigellae, campylobacters, and other specific intestinal pathogens affect hospitals as they do any community, with the added complication of the relatively low resistance of the patients.

Epidemic gastro-enteritis in infants, due to infection with certain specific serotypes of *Escherichia coli*, is a unique situation in hospital units where numbers of neonates or infants of under 2 years are nursed together. Severe acute diarrhoea can spread rapidly from child to child via the hands and clothes of the nursing and other staff.

SOURCES OF INFECTIOUS ORGANISMS

Infections may be exogenous, which means that they may result from an invasion of organisms into the body causing infection in a wound or burn, in the lung or in the urine or even generally throughout the body, or they may be endogenous, which means that the infection is caused by organisms which are already part of the flora of the body.

In hospital, simple exogenous infections are comparatively rare apart from those such as childhood fevers which may occur coincidentally as epidemics in the wards. Only a small number of infections of wounds, for example, can be shown to be due to direct contamination by organisms from the air or from unsterile dressings or instruments. The vast majority of hospital patients if infected are infected by organisms which have already colonized them and which have become part of the flora of their body.

Some organisms are long standing members of the body's flora. They are not characterized by especial virulence and are comparatively sensitive to antibiotic agents. Others, however, have colonized the body during hospitalization, replacing the original flora or adding to it. They are relatively more likely to cause infection, the infection may more often be severe and the organisms are more resistant to antibiotic therapy.

The colonization of the body with hospital organisms is an inexorable process and can be shown to progress steadily with each day of hospitalization. It is greatly influenced by the use of antibiotics, especially those with a broad spectrum which destroy the sensitive normal flora and open the way for the generally resistant invaders which may colonize the patient from other patients, from hospital staff, and from the environment.

The patient's skin and nose may be colonized with hospital staphylococci perhaps from the noses and skin of hospital staff who innocently carry them, from the dust of the ward where staphylococci survive well, from blankets during bed-making or during wound dressings. These staphylococci may well during surgery be introduced to wounds or other tissues. Group A, β-haemolytic streptococci are more directly spread in premature baby nurseries or in burns units where they can cause serious sepsis following colonization from the throats and noses of staff. The bowel flora of hospital patients is easily altered, especially following oral antibiotic therapy. Resistant Gram-negative bacilli, especially klebsiella and pseudomonas spp., are found and in extreme cases the normal bowel organisms may be repaced by resistant staphylococci or candida causing serious enteritis. Small babies may be colonized by specific entero-pathogenic serotypes of *Escherichia coli* and suffer infantile gastro-enteritis. The spread of bowel organisms to the skin of the perineum, hips, thighs and buttocks means that wound sepsis in these areas as well as in bowel surgery is due to infection with Gram-negative bacilli or with clostridia and bacteroides in many cases. The urinary tract is often infected in surgery or in catheterization with the organisms of the urethra and urethral meatus. Intensive care and prolonged cardiac, renal and neuro-surgery have necessitated the use of a wide variety of life support apparatus, vascular catheters, ventilators, humidifiers, and dialysers. These present ideal conditions for colonization with Gram-negative bacilli, especially *Pseudomonas aeruginosa*, which then pass to other patients and are particularly difficult to eradicate.

PREVENTIVE MEASURES

The effective control and prevention of hospital infection depends on action being taken not only to destroy the micro-organisms identified as causing it but to influence and diminish the factors which encourage them to thrive and spread, and to protect and reduce the availability of susceptible tissue which they colonize and damage.

The necessary action to achieve these ends must be agreed and accepted by medical, nursing and other staff and a representative "Control of Infection Committee" should be set up. It should secure agreement on a wide variety of measures including the following:

ward design and practice;
theatre design and practice;
sterilization and sterile supplies;
cleaning and disinfection;
antibiotic usage;
isolation of patients;
hospital hygiene;
special units;
staff health.

Ward Design and Practice

Design

Modern wards consist of arrangements of six, four or two bed units with several single-bed rooms which can be used to isolate the infectious or susceptible patient. Artificial ventilation is not necessary unless dictated by the climate. All surfaces, floors, walls, and ceilings should be smooth and washable. There should be a separate 'Dressings Room' or 'Procedures Cubicle', artificially ventilated, in which wound dressings, urethral catheterization, lumbar puncture or chest aspiration can be carried out rather than in the ward where traffic, bed-making and other activities disperse organism-bearing dust particles.

Practice

In the ward, as in any hospital area, the most important factors in the prevention of the transfer of infection are the attitude, behaviour and discipline of the staff. All must follow the rules of asepsis and hygiene, not just the most junior nurse but the most senior surgeon also.

Some hospital organisms colonize patients more or less directly from staff or other patients, especially the *Streptococcus pyogenes* and *Staphylococcus aureus*. In some few selected situations it may be necessary to ensure that staff are not carrying organisms particularly dangerous to their patients. Staff about to work in burns units and premature baby units may be screened for carriage of the streptococci in their throats or noses and treated by oral penicillin if positive. Hospital staff have a high rate of nasal carriage of staphylococci of phage types particularly associated with antibiotic resistance and it may be worth screening staff working with immunologically compromised patients and treating those with particular undesirable strains with local antiseptics.

Most infection in hospital is due to organisms carried in and on the patient and the utmost care must be taken to make sure that these organisms are not allowed to gain access to or flourish in susceptible tissues.

Respiratory infection can often be prevented by active physiotherapy to promote coughing and chest drainage after operation and anaesthesia. Pre-operative physiotherapy and stopping smoking for as long as possible before and after surgery are also helpful. When patients require mechanical aid to respiration they are especially vulnerable. Gram-negative bacilli, especially *Pseudomonas aeruginosa*, can be found widely in moist situations such as reservoirs in apparatus and in sinks and drains in units such as intensive care wards. All apparatus should be cleaned, dried, disinfected, and sterilized, and water in reservoirs should be changed daily.

Urinary tract infection in hospital is often associated with surgical interference or catheterization. It is important that urinary flow is maintained. Catheterization should only be carried out if therapeutically necessary, never merely to obtain a specimen. If it must be done it requires aseptic technique and chlorhexidene cream should be used on the catheter. Indwelling catheters should drain into a closed vessel or plastic bag with non-return valves to prevent back-flow to the bladder. Gastro-intestinal infection may occur in hospital. Food poisoning should not occur if there is good hygiene. Epidemic gastro-enteritis in infants may be due to specific enteropathogenic serotypes of *Escherichia coli* or rotaviruses (Chapter VIII). Even strict hygiene and barrier nursing can be ineffective in checking the spread of these very infectious conditions. It is necessary also to isolate the unit, stop admissions and transfers and discharge home all babies who are sufficiently well and who do not have infant siblings at home. The unit should be cleaned and disinfected before being re-opened.

Operating Theatre Design and Practice

Design

Good design should provide an area separated from external contamination so as to allow exposure of susceptible tissue in operative procedures. The suite is divided into 'clean' and 'dirty' areas. Within the clean area is the operating room, the scrub area where the staff wash their hands and don theatre gowns and gloves, the anaesthetic room, and the instrument preparation room. The dirty area comprises the arrival corridor, the changing rooms, and the dirty utility room where instruments and linen are gathered after operation. Simple but controlled flow of goods, patients and staff should be established between dirty and clean areas so that a 'red line' can be drawn between them. Staff should arrive by a dirty corridor and pass from it into appropriate changing rooms. When in theatre clothes and boots they should pass into a clean corridor and the operating suite. Any facilities or restrooms required should be on the clean side of the red line. Patients should be brought to theatre by ward porters on clean beds or trolleys in clean sheets and gowns and taken over from the red line by 'clean' porters. Theatre ventilation is by filtered air, humidified and temperature controlled. Air input and extraction should be so related that a pressure gradient exists in the theatre suite downwards from the theatre and instrument preparation rooms to the anaesthetic and scrub rooms to the clean corridor and changing rooms and finally to the dirty utility room and dirty corridor. Air changes by the system remove air-borne organisms dispersed from the theatre staff. More sophisticated air curtains and laminar flow systems are also available.

Practice

Skin preparation

Preparation of the skin of the patient for operation should begin if possible 1 or 2 days in advance of the operation by thorough washing followed by anointing the skin of the operation area with an iodophor preparation twice daily. In theatre the operation area should be rigorously anointed with iodine 1% in 70% alcohol or chlorhexidene 0.5% in 70% alcohol. The incision area must be free of hair.

Hand preparation

The preparation of the hands of operating staff is a matter of personal choice but approved methods include:

i) washing with 4% iodophor preparation (Betadine);

ii) washing with 4% chlorhexidene preparation (Hibiscrub);

iii) washing with 3% hexachlorophene preparation (Phisohex or Sterzac).
This last should be used repeatedly to achieve a cumulative antibacterial effect.

Staff Clothing

Staff should don theatre pyjamas or dresses, gowns, masks, and gloves. The clothing should be cotton or of specially woven fabric with a small pore size to cut down contamination from particles from the operator's body. Masks may be of paper or woven fabric. Paper masks must be discarded after one operation and any mask must be discarded if wet. Caps should cover all the hair and beards must be totally covered.

Sterilization and Sterile Supply Service

Methods of sterilization are dealt with in Chapter XV. In a modern hospital all surgical instruments, dressings and theatre linen should be sterile. Apparatus and materials difficult to sterilize due to heat sensitivity or problems of construction should be free of harmful organisms as far as possible. Responsibility for sterilization and sterile supply should be in the hands of a centralized sterile supply service.

Antibiotic Policy

The use of antibiotics is reviewed in Chapter XVI. It is vital that all prescribers of antibiotics are in agreement on what antibiotics may be used in given circumstances, as the hospital environment is not divisible. The individual needs of the patient may be paramount but the prevention of the establishment of resistant organisms in the environment is to the benefit of all. From this point of view antibiotics used in therapy should be:

a) used only where necessary;
b) effective;
c) narrow spectrum;
d) bactericidal;
e) in common use in the hospital;
f) continued for a definite period only;
g) if new and little used, given to the patient in isolation.

Prophylactic use of antibiotics should be controlled and used only in agreed circumstances (Chapter XVI).

Isolation

The separation of pathogenic organisms from susceptible tissue is a cardinal aim in control of infection.

The highly infectious patient

For the protection of other patients, anyone with serious infection must be removed from the environment. Measles, wound sepsis or intestinal infection for example can be a serious risk.

Barrier nursing

The patients are nursed in an open ward with careful handling to avoid the passage of organisms from them on attendants' hands or clothes or on other articles. It does nothing to stop air-borne organisms.

Side ward isolation

Barrier nursing techniques are still employed and the spread of air-borne organisms is diminished. A simple extract window fan will draw air from the ward to the patient. The patient has the advantage of remaining under the care of the ward staff.

Isolation units and hospitals

Classical infections such as diphtheria, poliomyelitis or typhoid, or serious intractable wound infections, should be removed to isolation in Infectious Diseases Hospitals or Units. Patients with infectious tuberculosis should be removed to a tuberculosis unit.

The highly susceptible patient

Those whose ability to resist infection is reduced must be protected from invasion and colonization by infectious organisms. They should be segregated from their fellow patients in protective isolation and handled using techniques of 'Reverse Barrier Nursing'. In this every effort should be made to avoid introducing harmful micro-organisms to the patient. It is required for example in leukaemia, marrow aplasia, uraemia and in immunosuppression and steroid treatment. The very old and very young, especially the premature, also need protection, as do the seriously injured or burned.

A simple ward single room may be used together with reverse barrier nursing. Again, a window fan may be sufficient with the flow from outdoors into the single room and thence to the ward environment.

Higher degrees of protection are sometimes required in specially designed clean units. Here the air is filtered, the unit is at positive pressure and all articles brought to the unit can be sterilized, even the patient's food. The staff can be screened for carriage of particularly pathogenic organisms and should wear gowns, masks and gloves.

It is of course vital that the two types of isolation 'Infectious' and 'Protective' are entirely separated one from the other.

Hospital Hygiene

This should be controlled by agreed policies on:
cleaning and disinfecting the environment;
laundering of linen;
handling of food, dishes, and cutlery;
disposal of rubbish.

Cleaning and disinfecting

The general environment should be socially clean and greater effort should be spent on disinfection of areas such as theatres, wards, treatment rooms and special units as appropriate.

A limited number of chemical agents will suffice to meet all the needs for disinfection of the general environment. Some details of their characteristics will be found in Chapter XVI. Antiseptics for use on the skin of patients and staff are discussed on page 188.

Laundering and linen

Normal laundering, properly carried out in modern machines, will clean and disinfect clothing, bedclothes and towels. Linen contaminated or fouled should be separately bagged and carefully treated. Linen from patients positive for infectious hepatitis is subjected to 93°C for 10 minutes in the laundering process or autoclaved. Disposable linen may be used.

Food, dishes, and cutlery

Food

The service of food is now usually centralized in large kitchens, and dishes and cutlery are returned there for centralized washing and disinfection. The degree of centralization imposes the responsibility for scrupulous care to avoid food-borne infection on a large scale.

Milk feeds

Infant milk feeds are almost entirely purchased from commercial sources and can be stored at room temperature. Local preparation is rare but should be carried out with scrupulous cleanliness using boiled water and powdered milk. Such feeds are subjected to free steaming at 100–105°C. This is not sterilization and spores of *Bacillus cereus* survive. The milk feeds must be stored in a refrigerator. Sterile disposable teats should be used. Milk banks in which human milk is collected from donors, subsequently to be given to babies, present problems of handling. When milk is pooled or provided for unrelated babies it must be pasteurized which unfortunately may inactivate maternal antibodies. Milk provided for a mother's own baby may be collected with scrupulous care, stored at 4°C and used fresh.

Rubbish disposal

This requires that all forms of waste for disposal should be removed from the environment with minimum contamination of it. Sealed plastic bags and sacks are usually colour coded for different forms of waste and incineration is usually employed to destroy rubbish safely.

Sharp needles and instruments for disposal should be dropped after use into plastic containers strong enough to protect those handling them from injury. Contaminated or infectious material should remain under responsible supervision until destroyed.

Special Units and Hazards

Intensive care units

The patients in such units often have reduced resistance and require mechanical assistance to breathe, to clear their airways, to pass urine and to feed. Their natural defences are bypassed and the most scrupulous attention must be paid to asepsis and good practice to avoid introducing infection to them even when life saving action is going on. There should be a strict protocol for cleaning and disinfecting respirators, ventilators, humidifiers and similar apparatus with particular care of humidifiers and reservoirs which breed *Pseudomonas aeruginosa*.

Haemodialysis and renal units

Patients with renal failure have low resistance and are liable to be infected by the virus of serum hepatitis and particularly liable to become carriers of the hepatitis B surface antigen (HB_sA_g positive). Patients must be screened before admission and treated separately quite outside the unit if positive. Staff should be screened before being allowed to work in these units and patients and staff must be screened at intervals of 1–3 months. Especial careful technique to avoid contamination with blood or excretions should be practised and specimens from patients treated as dangerous and specially marked. Anti HB globulin can be used to protect staff in case of accident.

Staff Health and Immunization

There should be a staff occupational health service with suitable premises and staff.

Immunization should be given against poliomyelitis, tetanus, tuberculosis and rubella as indicated and typhoid, anthrax, diphtheria or other infections in specific cases of risk.

All staff should have a chest x-ray on appointment. Thereafter every 3 years is sufficient except for those at special risk of tuberculosis in wards or laboratories, who should have annual x-rays. Staff working in neonatal and paediatric units should also have annual chest x-rays because of the high susceptibility of those in their care.

CHAPTER XV

Sterilization and Disinfection in Hospitals

INTRODUCTION

An important consideration in the care of patients in hospital is that no infection should be introduced to them by any agent used upon them or from the environment in which they are treated.

It is therefore necessary that steps be taken to reduce, or better still, to eliminate from the environment the micro-organisms in it, especially those which may be harmful to the patient. This is particularly true when an object, instrument or substance is going to come into close contact with or penetrate the patient. Every effort must be applied to achieve sterilization or disinfection.

DEFINITIONS

Sterilization is ridding an object or substance of all forms of microbial life including bacterial spores.

Disinfection is ridding an object or substance of pathogenic organisms in the vegetative phase.

METHODS OF STERILIZING AND DISINFECTING

The major methods used are summarized in Table XV.1 with an indication as to whether they can, properly applied, achieve sterilization or only disinfection.

Any method depends for its success on the applied agent actually reaching and affecting the micro-organisms concerned. It must do so for a sufficient time. In a method relying on heat, the correct temperature must be achieved and additionally in moist-heat methods the water or the steam must itself penetrate to the micro-organisms. In irradiation there must be ionic penetration. In chemical methods the concentration of the agent and the time of exposure must together be sufficient. The 'pore

Table XV.1 Practical Methods of Sterilization and Disinfection

	Method	Time of exposure	Sterilization/ Disinfection
Moist Heat	1. Water at 80°C	10 minutes	Disinfection
	2. Boiling water	10 minutes	Disinfection
	3. Steam at 73°C	20 minutes	Disinfection
	4. Steam at 134°C	3 minutes	Sterilization
Dry Heat	Hot air at 160°C	1 hour	Sterilization
Gas	Ethylene oxide 55°C	1 hour	Sterilization
	Low temperature steam and formaldehyde 73°C	2 hours	Sterilization
Irradiation	Gamma-rays, 2.5 megarad	—	Sterilization

size' of a filter will determine which organisms can pass when filtration is the method used.

In every method employed, success also considerably depends on the microbial load or challenge with which the agent has to deal. It is absolutely vital that this be reduced as far as possible before the process is applied. Cleaning must come before sterilization or disinfection. Avoidance of contamination in manufacture or handling will make sterilization easier and more certain.

Physical Methods

Heat

The application of heat is the simplest and most readily controlled method of both disinfection and sterilization. It may be applied as dry heat or moist heat.

Dry heat

The killing effect of dry heat depends on the oxidation of the substance of the organism. This takes place at relatively high temperatures and both spores and vegetative organisms are killed. The methods used are:

Incineration

This is used for safe disposal by burning or for sterilizing by flaming.

Hot air ovens

Objects to be sterilized are placed in an electric oven at 160°C for 1 hour with the air in the oven circulated by an internal fan. The method damages materials such as paper, cloth, rubber and almost all plastics and its use is limited to a small number of instruments. Instruments may be processed in air tight metal containers and thereafter stored sterile in them indefinitely.

Moist heat

Hot water or steam can be used to kill by coagulation of the protein of the cell wall, at a lower temperature and in a shorter time than required using dry heat.

Pasteurization in water

This is a form of disinfection at a temperature low enough not to damage heat sensitive material or apparatus. Ths instrument is cleaned, placed unwrapped in a waterbath and a temperature of 80°C is held for 10 minutes. A thermometer and thermostat are required. Spores are not killed.

Boiling in water

The disinfection is at 100°C so that damage may be more likely. A thermostat and thermometer are not required. Spores are not killed.

Pasteurization in steam

Exposure to steam in an autoclave at sub-atmospheric pressure is a very effective method of disinfecting heat sensitive instruments: 73°C for 20 minutes achieves disinfection and in addition a large proportion of spores will be killed.

Sterilization by steam at above atmospheric pressure

This is the most commonly used method of sterilizing instruments, dressings, linen, and many pieces of apparatus used in hospital.

    1) 'Instrument Autoclave'. These are still used in isolated theatre suites to sterilize simple instruments and articles with all their surfaces exposed

and unwrapped. No linen or paper wrapping and no gowns, sheets or dressings can be processed. This is because sterilization by steam depends on actual contact between the steam and the organisms to be killed. Nothing must prevent the total removal of residual air from the autoclave and its contents or interfere with total penetration of pure steam to all surfaces. These simple autoclaves depend for the removal of air from the chamber on its displacement downwards through the chamber drain by the lighter incoming steam which fills the chamber from the top. Pure steam at 305 KPa absolute (30 lbs/sq in above atmospheric pressure) has a temperature of 134°C and this is held for 3 minutes after which the steam is drawn out and air readmitted through a filter. As the unwrapped instruments are immediately recontaminated when the door is opened, these autoclaves can only be used in the clean areas of operating suites. They produce heat and noise and misuse the time of skilled staff and are little used now in modern hospitals.

2) 'Porous Load Autoclave'. This apparatus differs from the Instrument Autoclave in one important aspect. Downward displacement is replaced in a pre-vacuum period by 'pulsing' with five or six alternate vacuums and steam pulses or flushing by continuous vacuum and steam infusion to remove all the air from both chamber and contents. Linen, cloth, paper and instruments and apparatus wrapped in these permeable materials can be sterilized by exposure to pure steam. This means that sterilization can be carried out in a Central Sterile Supply Department. Instruments, apparatus and linen can be removed protected and still sterile at the end of the cycle, and stored subsequently until required. Sterilizing is at 134°C at 305 KPa absolute in pure steam for 3 minutes.

Monitoring of autoclaves

It is impossible to prove that any process has sterilized the load of articles treated by examining samples from it. Even if the entire load is tested to destruction any tests applied cannot take account of the variety of conditions of incubation required to grow each possible remaining contaminant.

Estimation of the effect of a process must be by showing that certain measurable parameters have been met in certain pre-determined sites. An enormous weight of experience can be built up in practice to indicate that when these parameters have been met there has been no evidence that contaminant organisms have survived.

Physical parameters are the most reliable. Autoclaves should indicate and record pressure and temperature. Sensors should be in both the chamber drain and in devices from which it is difficult to extract air and into which it is difficult to introduce steam. These devices simulate conditions in bulky wrapped packs or within narrow lumina of instruments. There should be facilities to draw full vacuum and estimate the leak rate into the machine.

Chemical parameters consists of impregnated tapes, 'autoclave tape' or fluid in glass ampoules, e.g. Browne's autoclave tubes. Autoclave tape is the basis of the Bowie Dick test in which a pack of folded towels wrapped in linen is used to test air removal and penetration of steam. Diagonal stripes on the adhesive tape stuck on the centre towel change from pale to black on exposure to steam dependent on time and temperature. The test is minutely defined and must be carried out exactly. Browne's tubes may be scattered in a load as they are small cheap ampoules. The chemical contained alters from red to green on exposure to appropriate temperature for appropriate time. The tubes do not distinguish between dry heat and moist heat.

Microbiological monitors are least satisfactory although killing micro-organisms is what is actually at issue. Test pieces consist of heat resistant spores dried on to filter paper or aluminium foil. There are considerable variations in viable numbers, heat resistance, germination, and recovery however carefully the tests are prepared and subsequently cultured. Results are of course only available after an arbitrary period of growth, 10–14 days in defined media and conditions, and can only be retrospective in most cases.

Radiation

Sterilization by exposure to ionizing radiation is widely used in industry to process disposable items but does not have a place in hospitals. Gamma-rays are best employed in a dose of 25 k Gray (2.5 Mrad) and sterilization is achieved provided there is penetration. It is important that the microbial challenge be kept as low as possible by good manufacturing practice.

Ultraviolet radiation depends on the bactericidal effect of rays of about 250 nm. These are produced by mercury vapour lamps. They have considerable disadvantage in that they can be damaging to skin, eyes and other tissues and the lamps must therefore be shielded. They are only useful to sterilize exposed surfaces as they do not penetrate at all well and their effect is relatively poor against viruses. A constant check on the emission of the lamps must be made, as their performance decreases quite quickly. Their use is generally limited to small enclosed areas such as laboratory inoculation cabinets when not in use. Ultraviolet light has been used also to sterilize water in specially designed apparatus.

Filtration

Filtration is a method of removing organisms from a fluid or gas which can be passed through the small pores and passages of a filter. It is not necessary to kill the organisms to achieve sterilization. All that is needed is a filter with the capability of holding back organisms of given sizes while allowing the gas or fluid to pass. The most difficult organisms to remove are the smallest and a division can be made into filters which remove only the bacteria, which are relatively large, and those which will also remove viruses. Total removal including viruses is referred to as absolute filtration. Filtration of air is used in operating theatres and other clean areas (Chapter XV), and filtration of fluids is practised in pharmacies and laboratories to render safe those drugs and infusions or laboratory media which cannot be heated, irradiated or chemically treated. It should be noted that filtration also removes the actual bodies of the organisms and in this respect may be superior to methods which kill but leave the substance of the organisms behind to act as impurities and on infusion into a patient cause pyrogenic reactions.

Chemical methods

Disinfection and sometimes sterilization can be achieved by a variety of chemical agents. Many are fluids and have to be applied to the apparatus or instrument to be processed, or these have to be immersed in the fluid. Most fluid agents act by a chemical reaction with the micro-organisms and any other proteins present and it is essential that cleaning precede the process and that as little foreign protein as possible be present so as to avoid using up the chemical in useless and unnecessary activity. Chemical methods are not as reliable nor as effective as methods employing heat and they cannot be so reliably monitored. This is also true of the two main chemical gas methods used in this country to try to achieve sterilization of instruments and apparatus which are heat labile and which will not withstand sterilization by heat. These are exposure to ethylene oxide gas and exposure to low temperature steam and formaldehyde. Both achieve their effect by reactions with the carboxyl, amino, hydroxyl and sulphydryl groups of protein and probably by binding reactions with the nucleic acid.

Ethylene oxide

This gas is an extremely effective penetrating bactericidal agent. It is unfortunately toxic, explosive and inflammable and on these grounds is relatively little used in Britain although more popular in America and Europe. It also has been condemned as ineffective in the presence of dirt, serum or salt.

For safety it is usually employed carried in an inert gas vehicle, such as CO_2 or one of the rare gases, at a less than explosive mixture e.g. 15% ethylene oxide and 85% CO_2 at 55°C and a relative humidity of 80% for a holding period of 1 hour. Problems of subsequent elution of the toxic gas from processed materials into body tissues or fluids mean that the items processed which are often of plastic should not be used until after an airing-off period of 7 days and they must be stored in a well ventilated area.

The ethylene oxide process cannot be measured physically with any of the certainty of sterilization by heat. It is very dependent on the successful penetration of the load by the gas in the presence of a reasonable relative humidity and the absence of protective factors such as salt or serum. Biological test pieces must be depended on instead and are much less satisfactory.

Low temperature steam and formaldehyde (LTSF)

In Britain this is the method of general choice to process heat sensitive items in hospital. It uses a combination of both physical and chemical processes. Exposure is to steam at sub-atmospheric pressure within a sterilizer chamber, with in this case the addition of a chemical agent, formaldehyde gas. Monomeric formaldehyde gas and dry saturated steam at the chosen temperature of 73°C must contact all surfaces to be sterilized.

The actual cycle used in the process is still a matter of choice. Emphasis may be on exposure first to formaldehyde gas in considerable concentration followed by exposure to steam, or alternatively a long series of pulses of steam may be admitted to the chamber with low concentrations of formaldehyde used. In either case the process is carried out in an autoclave with the chamber surrounded by a jacket heated by steam or water to slightly above the chamber temperature. Articles can be processed enclosed in porous wrapping or paper bags and have the same shelf life as those autoclaved at 134°C. An advantage of the method is that the temperature of 73°C for 2 hours will itself kill many vegetative organisms which may be in situations where steam and formaldehyde have failed to penetrate. There are no dangers of fire and explosion and the system, which is relatively cheap to run, will deal with all but a very few heat sensitive items. There is little problem with residual toxicity.

Liquid chemical agents

A wide variety of chemical agents available in liquid form act as disinfectants or in some cases sterilizers in the environment, where they can be used on instruments, furniture, walls, and floors as appropriate. In addition some chemicals can be used to reduce the microbial load on the skin of the patient or on the surgeon's or nurse's hands. These antiseptics have to be of course relatively non-damaging in nature and it should be noted that there is no way of sterilizing the skin without its damage or destruction.

Out of the large number available it is only necessary to consider a few which best meet the needs of different situations occurring in the wards, theatres and departments of the hospital. An ideal chemical would have the following qualities:

> wide activity against all microorganisms including spores;
> rapid activity, killing at once;
> a cleaning and detergent action;
> no toxic or damaging action on people or materials;
> continued activity in the presence of foreign protein and dirt;
> resistance to inactivation by soaps, detergents, and plastics.

Regrettably, no single agent possesses all these qualities, so that it is necessary to select the one most appropriate in the circumstances accepting its deficiencies. The agents to be considered are the following: alcohol, formaldehyde, glutaraldehyde, hypochlorite, iodine, soluble phenolics, quaternary ammoniums, and diguanides. Their activity against Gram-positive and Gram-negative organisms, *M. tuberculosis* and the spore bearers varies very considerably.

In addition to the inactivation of chemicals by protein which has been already mentioned, they may also be inactivated by soap, detergents, both cationic and anionic, and by plastic or other materials.

Alcohol

Methyl or iso-propyl alcohol are used as 70% in water. Pure alcohol is not effective. The advantage of alcohol is its fast action, its de-greasing activity which is useful in cleaning the skin and other greasy surfaces, and its subsequent evaporation and disappearance. These qualities make it the basis of skin antiseptics where with the addition of iodine or chlorhexidine it can kill quickly and widely. It can also be used for example for wiping down the tops of previously clean metal trolleys. It is not easily inactivated but it does not kill spores.

Formaldehyde

This is an extremely powerful but very toxic and damaging agent. In addition to its use in the LTSF process, Formalin A.R. containing 40% formaldehyde w/v can be boiled off to fumigate laboratories, inoculation cabinets and areas contaminated by serious infection. Its use in wards and isolation rooms is of dubious value, but as the process requires that the room be sealed, left for 24 hours and subsequently aired and cleaned down, the whole ritual has value in preventing cross infection. Formaldehyde will kill spores.

Glutaraldehyde

Of the same family, this agent also is very powerful, toxic, and damaging. It is used in 2% solution (Cidex) which is activated in an alkaline buffer at pH 8.0 but thereafter has a relatively short active life of 2 weeks. Longer acting formulations are available but it is doubtful if these are advantageous. It will kill all organisms including spores in a few hours provided the fluid has access to them. Some expensive instruments including fibre-optic endoscopes can only be sterilized by immersion in glutaraldehyde but it should be remembered that thorough pre-cleaning including washing through patent lumina is an essential part of the process and that the glutaraldehyde has to be washed off completely before the instruments can be used.

Hypochlorite

This very powerful chlorinating and oxidizing agent will kill all organisms including spores but unfortunately is very easily inactivated by protein and by cationic detergents. This is a serious limitation to its use which must be restricted to clean surfaces. It is widely employed in bleaching and scouring baths and wash basins (Domestos, Chloros) and in clean surfaces in food preparation (Kirbychlor) where it can be washed off afterwards and before use. As 'Milton' it is a popular method of sterilizing washed baby feeding bottles. It is used in discard jars especially in virology laboratories and it is very widely used in swimming baths and in the disinfection of water supplies.

Iodine

This agent is most useful in skin preparation as a 1% solution in 70% alcohol. It is widely effective and will kill spores after sufficient exposure. There is some danger of allergy to it but this is less with improved iodophor preparations which are used undiluted (Betadine or Povidine Iodine).

Soluble Phenolics

These solutions are very widely used for general cleaning in hospital particularly in dirty conditions in the presence of organic matter. The resistance of these compounds to inactivation or quenching by organic matter is a very important factor in their use but it should be remembered that some plastics will inactivate them. They will disinfect faeces or pus and can be used on dirty floors and for steeping foul linen. Examples of commercial products include 'Clearsol' and 'Hycolin'.

Quaternary ammonium compounds (QACs)

These compounds have a good cleaning action and low toxicity and are not damaging. They can be used for cleaning the skin or the environment but it should be remembered that they are almost totally ineffective against Gram-negative bacilli and spores other than by washing them away. Solutions easily become contaminated and can actually themselves contaminate rather than disinfect. Cetrimide and benzalkonium chloride are commonly used QACs.

Diguanides

These agents have considerable effect on Gram-positive organisms even in very low concentration and some effect on Gram-negative bacilli but none on spores. They are usually employed with alcohol as a skin preparation or with a quaternary ammonium as a cleansing disinfectant. Chlorhexidine 0.05% with 0.5% cetrimide (Cetavlon) is marketed as 'Savlon Hospital Concentrate' for environmental cleaning and Chlorhexidine 0.5% in 70% alcohol is marketed as 'Hibitane' for skin preparation. Chlorhexidine can also be used in antiseptic creams and in soaps and creams for hand washing.

Testing chemical agents

Almost all testing of disinfectants is the responsibility of the developer and manufacturer and of a few specialized laboratories. Once the activity of a disinfectant in different conditions is established and understood it should be necessary to practice only to confirm that in the actual circumstances in which it is being employed at the time that the disinfectant is potent and has not been inactivated or contaminated.

Sterilization in industry

Many plastic items are provided already sterilized by the manufacturer. These are intended to be used once and then disposed of. The decision as to whether an item should be regarded as disposable is not only made on economic grounds, i.e. that it costs more to wash and re-sterilize it than to replace it. More important may be its ability to allow and withstand repeated sterilization by one method or re-sterilization by a different method. Many plastics are altered by sterilization and will deteriorate further if re-processed. For example irradiation of polyvinyl chloride must not be followed by exposure to ethylene oxide as toxic ethylene chlorhydrin is formed. For all these reasons, therefore, articles marketed as disposable should not be re-used.

CHAPTER XVI

Antibiotic and Chemotherapy

GENERAL ASPECTS OF ANTIBIOTIC USAGE

Although quinine had been used for the treatment of malaria since the early 17th century and the value of arsenical compounds in syphilis was demonstrated by Ehrlich in 1909, the first major advance in chemotherapy came in 1935 when German research workers produced prontosil which in the body liberates a sulphonamide. This substance was rapidly shown to be highly effective against β-haemolytic streptococci. It is important to remember that prior to that time nothing could be done to help a patient with such an infection and tragic deaths occurred in previously healthy young people; streptococcal puerperal sepsis was a particularly dreaded complication of childbirth.

Although penicillin had been discovered by Fleming in 1929, its therapeutic value was first demonstrated by Florey and his colleagues at Oxford in 1940 and from this work arose the whole of modern chemotherapy as we now know it.

The term 'antibiotic' has generally been reserved for antibacterial substances produced by micro-organisms, and indeed it was the recognition of the importance of inhibition of one micro-organism by another that influenced early work on penicillin. The term 'chemotherapeutic substance' may be used both for antibiotics and for synthetic compounds. However, many antibiotics may now be synthesized and the distinction, in everyday usage, of these terms is now blurred.

Following the introduction of penicillin into clinical use, great efforts were made to find new antibiotics and these were generally discovered as products of organisms present in soil surveys; although other sources were sometimes fruitful, for example cephalosporins were first isolated from a sewage outfall off Sardinia and fusidic acid from monkey dung. The dates of discovery of some of the important antibiotics are: streptomycin 1944, chloramphenicol 1947, chlortetracycline 1948, cephalosporin 1948, erythromycin 1952, fusidic acid 1960, lincomycin 1962, and gentamicin 1963. Since 1963 the major advances that have occurred have been due to modifications of existing antibiotics, particularly manipulation of the penicillin nucleus and the cephalosporin nucleus. One consequence of this has been that modern antibiotic therapy may seem to be quite complex due to the large numbers of antibiotics available. Some of these may be apparently different but in reality closely related. It is important that medical students should attempt to have a reasonable knowledge of the major groups of antibiotics available to provide a basis for future rational prescribing. In the U.K. for example, antibiotics account for 15–20% of the drug bill of hospitals and at any one time 15% of hospital in-patients will be receiving antibiotic therapy. Informed and rational antibiotic prescribing is not only important in relation to individual patient care but also in relation to the prevention of development of antibiotic resistance by bacteria. There can be no doubt that levels of bacterial resistance in a community are directly related to levels of antibiotic usage. This occurs due to selection of a minority resistant population which can multiply in the presence of the antibiotic. Resistance may initially arise by mutation, but transfer of genetic material mediating antibiotic resistance between micro-organisms is probably of most importance. Transfer may be phage mediated (transduction) or may occur by conjugation. Transduction is particularly important in staphylococcal antibiotic resistance. Conjugation occurs between Gram-negative bacilli and when this happens not only may multiple antibiotic resistance be transferred, but this may occur between different species (Chapter I).

Although some degree of antibiotic resistance is seen wherever antibiotics are used, major problems arise for a number of particular reasons. In many countries antibiotics can be bought by the general population without a medical prescription. In addition laboratory facilities may be limited so that sensitivity testing of pathogens is impossible. Under these circumstances there is a great risk not only that specific pathogens become resistant but that the normal bowel flora of the human population may do so as well. This antibiotic resistance may subsequently be transferred to human pathogens and this is probably the mechanism whereby outbreaks of dysentery due to multiply antibiotic resistant organisms difficult to treat have occurred. Chloramphenicol resistant typhoid bacilli probably arose in the same way. Because plasmids transferred in conjugation may mediate multiple antibiotic resistance, the use of one antibiotic may select for resistance not only to that antibiotic but also to others when resistance to them is carried on the same plasmid.

Another area of difficulty is the use of antibiotics in animal husbandry. They may be used as food additives or given prophylactically or therapeutically. The first is the most important. Animal weight gain for the same food intake is increased if antibiotics are given and there are therefore good economic reasons for doing so. In some countries the antibiotics used as food additives are not those used in human medicine but even in these countries animals may receive such antibiotics for other reasons. The problem is most severe in intensively reared animals, particularly broiler chickens. If such animals carry multiply antibiotic resistant organisms, and this is commonly the situation, these may cause problems to the human population in two ways. Antibiotic resistant salmonellas may cause outbreaks of food poisoning in man. Although antibiotic therapy in food poisoning is not generally required, it may be necessary if septicaemia occurs and effective treatment may, therefore, be compromised. Another cause of difficulty is the transfer of multiply resistant coliforms to man. The ability of such organisms to establish in the bowel of man is a matter of debate but there is little doubt that if ingested they will be able to transfer antibiotic resistance to other organisms of the gut. These organisms provide a reservoir for transfer to human pathogens and if they give rise to infections, for example of the urinary tract, these may be difficult to treat.

The use of antibiotics by doctors, particularly in hospital, is also important. Units in which there has been high antibiotic usage, particularly if antibiotics have been used prophylactically or continued for long periods, tend to be those in which intractable outbreaks of antibiotic resistant infection occur. An outbreak occurring in such circumstances is likely to be serious and difficult to eradicate. This happens in intensive care units, special care baby units, neuro-surgical wards, and similar places and it is in these areas that the need for sensible policies in the use of antibiotics is particularly great.

PRINCIPLES TO BE CONSIDERED WHEN PRESCRIBING ANTIBIOTICS

Therapeutic use

When considering whether to prescribe an antibiotic and which one to use, a number of points should be considered.

It is essential, except in very unusual circumstances, to make a clinical diagnosis before commencing therapy. This may appear so obvious that it does not need saying, but the temptation to 'try an antibiotic' may be strong if the diagnosis is obscure. The consequences of partial and inadequate treatment of a disease such as subacute bacterial endocarditis may be very serious.

Having decided that infection is present, antibiotics should not be administered if the infection is trivial and will heal without antibiotics. Although antibiotics are as a group very safe drugs, there is no antibiotic in use which does not in a small number of patients give rise to side effects and these may be serious.

The next decision to be made is whether it is necessary to isolate the infecting organism. In hospital patients this should always be attempted and specimens should be taken before therapy is started. Treatment should not usually await laboratory results. In domicilary practice, where access to laboratory facilities may be more difficult and where the problems of nosocomial flora do not exist, many infections can reasonably be treated without laboratory aid. These include such things as uncomplicated urinary tract infection, upper respiratory tract infection, particularly in children, and the exacerbations of chronic bronchitis. As long as the limitations of such a policy are remembered, this may well be a satisfactory approach.

When laboratory results are obtained it may be necessary to change the antibiotic in use because antibiotic resistance has been reported. The laboratory report should give the sensitivity results of the infecting organism to a limited number of antibiotics which are likely to be useful in that clinical situation. It should also conform with the general policy of the hospital on the use of antibiotics.

When the laboratory report is available, the choice of antibiotic will then depend on a number of factors, but the over-riding considerations are efficacy and safety. The least toxic effective antibiotic should be chosen. However, the cost of the antibiotic and the route of administration should also be borne in mind, other things being equal.

With many antibiotics there is a choice of route of administration. Intravenous therapy may be necessary for severe life-threatening infections but oral therapy will be far preferable for less severe disease. It may on occasion be necessary to change the antibiotic after a period of therapy. This is not due to acquisition of resistance by the initial infecting organism during therapy which is not often seen, but is due to infection with a second organism. This is regularly seen in wound infection, when a staphylococcal infection may be replaced by a coliform organism resistant to the antibiotic being used. Repeat specimens should be taken.

There is little real evidence about the effectiveness of different antibiotic dosage regimen and the length of time for which treatment should be continued. In patients with an unimpaired immunological response antibiotic therapy is generally very effective, the antibiotic merely helping an effective immune system. However, in immunologically compromised patients even prolonged high dose therapy may fail.

The use of combinations of antibiotics is best avoided if possible. It is not often necessary; it increases the risk of toxic side effects and the cost of treatment. In a few circumstances, combined antibiotics may be needed. These include tuberculosis, where therapy with one antibiotic rapidly results in the appearance of resistant tubercle bacilli. Unlike most situations this is due to development of resistance by the original infecting organism. Combined therapy may also be used sometimes in sub-acute bacterial endocarditis, sometimes in mixed infections in which one antibiotic will not inhibit both organisms, and rarely in life-threatening infections in which the infecting organism is not known.

Prophylactic use

Prophylaxis is necessary in a number of situations. However, it does predispose to colonization of the patient with antibiotic resistant organisms and must be carefully controlled. Prophylaxis should be given generally for short periods so that this replacement of the sensitive flora does not occur. Some situations in which prophylaxis should be used are as follows:

In the prevention of recurrent attacks of rheumatic fever, penicillin is used to stop infection by *Streptococcus pyogenes*. This is one form of prophylaxis which is given for long periods. This is satisfactory because penicillin has a narrow spectrum of activity and *Streptococcus pyogenes* does not become resistant.

Dental treatment of patients with damaged heart valves from whatever cause should only be undertaken with antibiotic cover. Benzyl penicillin given intramuscularly 20 minutes before treatment, with oral penicillin for 1–2 days, is regularly used although some workers consider that the prevention of infections in patients wtih prosthetic heart valves may require antibiotics with a broad spectrum of activity (Chapter X).

Patients with wounds liable to develop gas gangrene should be given penicillin. This is most commonly needed in above knee amputations in diabetic patients.

Finally, some forms of surgery require prophylaxis. There is no doubt that the use of metronidazole which is effective against anaerobic organisms has revolutionized bowel surgery. Patients undergoing open heart surgery are also given prophylactic antibiotics. A number of regimen are in use, the most important factor being a short period of administration.

ANTIBIOTICS POLICIES

Because of the need to control antibiotic usage in hospitals, both for the benefit of the individual patients and the community as a whole, many hospitals have antibiotics policies. These generally provide for the regular use of a restricted range of antibiotics, with expensive, toxic, or particularly valuable antibiotics being reserved for occasional essential use. The policy often also includes advice on a 'best-buy' basis for the treatment of different types of infection, for example of the urinary tract or respiratory tract. This advice is based on the known antibiotic sensitivity patterns of commonly occurring pathogens in the hospital.

These policies are often useful to the junior doctor trying to find his way through what may appear to be a maze of antibiotics. It most certainly, however, does not absolve him from the responsibility of having a reasonable working knowledge of the antibiotics available and attempting to use them rationally.

LABORATORY ASPECTS OF ANTIBIOTIC THERAPY

Antiobiotic sensitivity is usually measured by looking for inhibition of growth of the organism in the presence of the antibiotic. Growth may be looked for on solid or in liquid media.

For most routine purposes disc sensitivity testing is adequate. Solid medium is used and a blotting paper disc containing a known amount of antibiotic is placed on a culture of the organism to be tested and a zone of inhibition looked for. This apparently simple technique gives rise to all sorts of problems. The size of the zone of inhibition will depend not only on the sensitivity of the organism to the antibiotic but also on the concentration of the antibiotic and the rate of diffusion which is affected by the molecular weight of the antibiotic, and the nature of the medium. The thickness of the medium will also affect the result, and if the antibiotic is allowed to diffuse before incubation this also will have an effect. It is desirable to control antibiotic sensitivity testing by putting an organism of known sensitivity on the same plate (Fig. XVI,1) and the zones of inhibition round the same disc to the two organisms can be compared. However, even with this control, results from different laboratories have differed. Although disc sensitivity testing is still almost universally used, attempts have been made to find other methods.

Antibiotic-containing
discs

Test
strain

Control
sensitive
strain

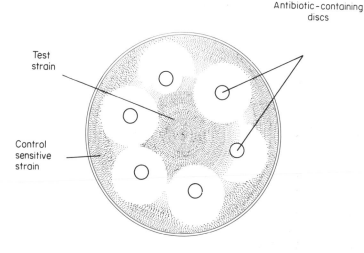

Figure XVI.1   Stokes plate used to compare the antibiotic sensitivity of an
unknown organism with that of a known sensitive strain

One such technique is the incorporation of increasing concentrations
of an antibiotic into a series of plates. About twenty organisms are
inoculated to each plate and the lowest level of antibiotic which inhibits
the growth of each organism is noted. This is known as end-point
titration antibiotic sensitivity testing.

A number of automated techniques are available. These involve
inoculating the test organisms into antibiotic-containing broth and
monitoring the turbidity of the fluid. A resistant organism will rapidly
produce a growth and the turbidity is automatically recorded. Such
equipment is gradually becoming more commonly used.

Determination of minimum inhibitory
and minimum bactericidal concentrations

In some situations accurate assessment of the sensitivity of an organism
is needed. In this case the minimum inhibitory concentration of antibiotics
to the organism is measured. This is the minimum level of the antibiotic
which inhibits multiplication of the organism and it is often measured by
making two-fold dilutions of the antibiotic inoculating the organism

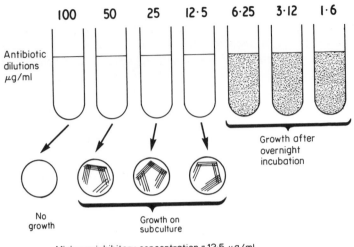

Figure XVI.2 A method of determining minimum inhibitory and minimum bactericidal concentrations

and looking after overnight incubation for growth of the organism (Fig. XVI,2).

From this test the minimum bactericidal concentration can also be measured. This is the minimum level of the antibiotic which actually kills the organism. This is done by subculturing the broths in which no growth has occurred to determine whether the bacteria are still viable and will grow when dilution of the antibiotic has taken place (Fig. XVI,2).

For some antibiotics the bacteriostatic and bactericidal levels are identical or very close (bactericidal antibiotics) but some antibiotics are never bactericidal even at high concentrations (bacteriostatic antibiotics).

MIC's (minimum inhibitory concentrations) and MBC's (minimum bactericidal concentrations) are usually required only in serious infection, particularly in immunocompromised patients, when it is important to ensure that the antibiotic regimen being used will be effective.

Antibiotic sensitivity testing in sub-acute bacterial endocarditis

There is one disease, sub-acute bacterial endocarditis, in which extensive laboratory investigations are essential to effective therapy. Initially, the infecting organism must be isolated if this is at all possible. The MBC of the organism to the antibiotic of choice (usually a penicillin) is determined. If it is expected that it will be possible to achieve this level in the blood stream, therapy should be started. Probenicid is added to reduce tubular excretion of the penicillin. After 1 or 2 days' therapy, blood is taken when the antibiotic level is at its lowest, i.e. immediately before the next dose is due. This can be examined in two ways. Either the antibiotic level can be determined — the method by which this is done will be described later — or doubling dilutions of the serum are inoculated with the infecting organism. After overnight incubation the dilution of serum which has killed the organism is determined. For practical purposes it is usual to aim at an antibiotic dosage which results in a 1 in 8 dilution of the pre-dose serum being bactericidal.

With some bacteria it is impossible to achieve this and combinations of antibiotics may be required. Classically penicillin and streptomycin have been used in the treatment of sub-acute bacterial endocarditis due to *Streptococcus faecalis*. Now many of the difficult infections seen are in patients with prosthetic heart valves. *Staph. albus* may be the infecting organism and the rather similar combination of ampicillin and gentamicin is more commonly used. If antibiotics are to be used in combination this must be looked at carefully, as the combination may be merely additive, or may be synergistic or antagonistic. A full chequer board titration may be done (Fig. XVI,4) but a useful result can be obtained more simply by making doubling dilutions of penicillin in a broth containing 2 μgm/ml streptomycin and comparing the MBC with that of penicillin alone.

Other methods of studying combinations of antibiotics involve the incorporation of the antibiotics into filter paper strips placed at right angles to each other and looking for patterns of growth (Fig. XVI,4). These techniques are interesting but not commonly used in routine laboratories.

Determination of serum antibiotic levels

There are a small number of antibiotics, of which gentamicin is the most commonly used, in which regular measurements of serum levels are necessary. Most antibiotics have a therapeutic level a long way below the toxic level so that the dosage need not be carefully controlled. In the case of gentamicin the toxic and therapeutic levels are close, that is the therapeutic index is low.

Gentamicin levels may be estimated to determine if toxic levels are being reached and if therapeutic levels have been achieved.

214

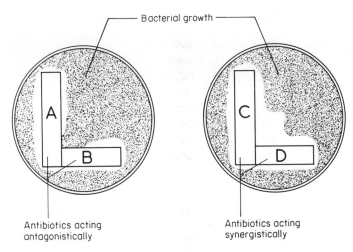

Figure XVI.3   Demonstration of antibiotic synergy and antagonism

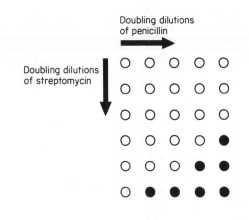

○ tubes of antibiotic-containing broth-no growth
● tubes of antibiotic-containing broth-growth

Figure XVI.4   A chequer board titration used to determine the efficacy of combinations of antibiotics

Toxic levels may occur in patients with impaired renal function who are given normal doses of gentamicin. The course of events is illustrated in Fig. XVI,5.

Blood should be taken immediately before gentamicin is given and if

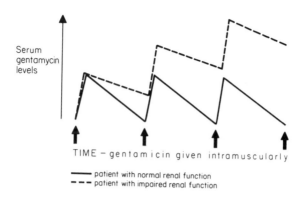

Serum gentamycin levels

TIME — gentamicin given intramuscularly

——— patient with normal renal function
--- patient with impaired renal function

Figure XVI.5   The 'staircase-effect' that occurs when gentamicin is given to a patient with impaired renal function

this pre-dose level begins to rise, the dosage should be reduced by increasing the interval between doses.

However, the commonest error in gentamicin prescribing is not the production of toxic effects but failure, due to inadequate dosage, to achieve a therapeutic level. It can be argued that all patients even without impaired renal function should have serum levels of gentamicin determined, in particular peak levels ½–1 hour after administration of the antibiotic.

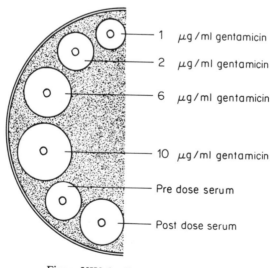

1   μg/ml gentamicin

2   μg/ml gentamicin

6   μg/ml gentamicin

10   μg/ml gentamicin

Pre dose serum

Post dose serum

Figure XIV.6   Gentamicin assay plate

The usual laboratory method of determining gentamicin levels is very simple and involves the estimation of the inhibition of a sensitive bacteria by the antibiotic in the patient's serum (Fig. XVI,6). Recently a number of rapid methods have been introduced and these are likely to come into more general use.

It is important to remember that the laboratory can give a great deal of assistance in antibiotic therapy. Treatment of sub-acute bacterial endocarditis and the administration of gentamicin should not be attempted without laboratory aid and indeed in many other situations very useful help can be given.

MODE OF ACTION

An effective antibiotic must be able to affect bacterial cells but not human ones and this is possible in the case of many antibiotics because of the major differences between procaryocytic and eucaryocytic organisms (Chapter I). Because one of the differences between the cells concerned is the possession by bacteria of a complex cell wall, some of the most effective antibiotics that we have act in this area. This is illustrated in Fig. XVI,7. The most important ones, penicillins and cephalosporins, act by preventing the final cross-linkage in the cell wall.

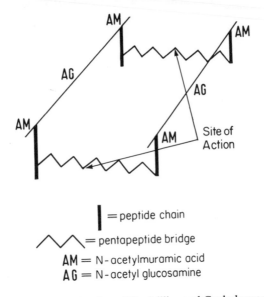

| = peptide chain
⋀⋀ = pentapeptide bridge
AM = N-acetylmuramic acid
AG = N-acetyl glucosamine

Figure XVI.7   Site of action of Penicillins and Cephalosporins

Another group of antibacterial agents with well-defined sites of action are the sulphonamides and trimethoprim. Because bacteria synthesizes folinic acid but man uses preformed folic or folinic acid present in the diet, the effect is highly selective for bacteria. The sequential action of sulphonamides and trimethroprim accounts for their synergy.

A number of other antibiotics act on protein synthesis. Streptomycin and other amino-glycosides cause the messenger RNA code to be misread and a wrong amino acid to be incorporated. Tetracycline interrupts the transport of amino acid to the ribosome. Transfer of the peptide chain is interrupted by chloramphenicol. Erythromycin affects both transfer and translocation.

From the above examples it might be expected that it would be possible to design antibiotics which act in particular ways. The major antibiotics in use have not been produced in this manner. However, interesting possibilities for the future exist in this type of approach.

MAJOR GROUPS OF ANTIBIOTICS
NOW REGULARLY IN CLINICAL USE

Penicillins

The penicillins are an extremely valuable group of antibiotics with extensive clinical usage. They are all predominantly bactericidal, and toxic side effects are rare but occur when large doses are given to patients with impaired renal function. Hypersensitivity reactions are more common and they occur with all penicillins. There may be immediate profound shock or serum sickness may develop later.

Alterations in the properties of the penicillins have been achieved by substitution of the side chain at A (Fig. XVI,8). A great diversity of penicillins is now available.

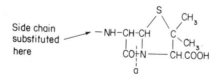

a = Site of action of β lactamases

Figure XVI.8

Benzyl penicillin (Penicillin G)

The structure of the side chain of benzyl penicillin is $\langle\!\!\!\bigcirc\!\!\!\rangle - CH_2\,CO -$

This was the first penicillin to be used clinically. It has to be given by intramuscular injection, has a short half life and a narrow spectrum of activity which includes *Streptococcus pyogenes*, the pneumococcus, non-penicillinase producing staphylococci, and neisseria. It is used in the treatment of streptococcal infections including tonsillitis, pneumococcal infections, particularly pneumonia and meningitis, gonorrhoea, and meningococcal meningitis.

Less soluble compounds of benzyl penicillin have been used to delay absorption and prolong the antibiotic effect. These include procaine penicillin which has some effect for up to 12 hours and benzathine penicillin which has an effect for several weeks. Benzathine penicillin is used in the prophylaxis of rheumatic fever. Benzyl penicillin and its insoluble salts are split at the position marked a in Fig. XVI,8 by lactamases produced by some bacteria. These β lactamases or penicillinases are an important mechanism of antibiotic resistance in a number of organisms, including many staphylococci.

Phenoxymethyl penicillin (penicillin V)

Side chain $\langle\!\!\!\bigcirc\!\!\!\rangle - O - CH_2 - CO-$

This is acid resistant and can be given by mouth. It has a similar but not identical spectrum of activity to benzyl penicillin and is β lactamase sensitive. It is used for mild streptococcal infections, particularly tonsillitis in children.

Ampicillin

Side chain $\langle\!\!\!\bigcirc\!\!\!\rangle - \underset{NH_2}{CH} - CO-$

Ampicillin is acid resistant and can be given by mouth. It is β lactamase sensitive and is less active against Gram-positive bacteria than benzyl penicillin but many times more active against Gram-negative bacilli. It is very widely used in the treatment of urinary tract infections, bronchitis, wound infections, and many other conditions. High dosage intravenous ampicillin is used in the treatment of haemophilus meningitis. Amoxycillin is a similar substance to ampicillin but is better absorbed and is more actively bactericidal. Pivampicillin and talampicillin are esters of ampicillin. They are completely absorbed and are then hydrolysed to liberate ampicillin. For this reason they produce higher blood levels than are attained with ampicillin which is incompletely absorbed.

Cloxacillin

Side chain

Cloxacillin is resistant to β lactamase, is acid stable and can be given by mouth. It is used in the treatment of staphylococcal infections due to β lactamase producing organisms. Flucloxacillin is similar but is better absorbed and is now generally used.

Carbenicillin

Side chain

This penicillin, unlike those previously described, is active against *Pseudomonas aeruginosa*. It is given parenterally; high dosage is needed for systemic infections and in this situation it is probably best combined with gentamicin.

Ticarcillin is generally similar to carbenicillin, but is rather more active. Azlocillin and piperacillin are also active against *Pseudomonas aeruginosa* including some strains resistant to carbenicillin and ticarcillin. They are ureido penicillins.

Mecillinam

Mecillinam is an amidino penicillin. It is active against Gram-negative organisms particularly proteus, serratia and klebsiellas and it has a synergistic effect with ampicillin. Mecillinam cannot be given by mouth but its ester pivmecillinam can.

Clavulanic acid

This is useful not because of its antibacterial activity but because it inhibits β lactamases. It can therefore be used in combination with a β lactamase sensitive penicillin to treat infections due to β lactamase producing organisms. Amoxycillin and clavulanic acid are used together, particularly in urinary tract infections.

Cephalosporins

In 1945 a fungus which produced cephalosporins was isolated from a sewage outfall off Sardinia. Cephalosporin C was a minority product of the mould and it is from this that the cephalosporins in use have been developed.

The structure of the cephalosporin ring is similar to that of penicillin (Fig. XVI,9). By substitution at A and B a range of products has been developed with varying properties. This is an area in which there have been many developments and the choice of the most suitable cephalosporin may be a difficult problem. Only some of the more commonly used cephalosporins and their main properties are given here. Cephalosporins are generally of very low toxicity. Some are nephrotoxic and sensitivity reactions occur in a small number of patients. There is some cross sensitization with penicillin.

The assessment of the best clinical role of the various cephalosporins is continuing. These compounds are generally active against a wide range of Gram-positive and Gram-negative organisms but there are important variations some of which are described below. In spite of this they do not feature amongst the antibiotics used as the first line of therapy in common conditions. The situation is complicated by the fact that the laboratory cannot give a 'cephalosporin' sensitivity, but the particular individual antibiotic to be used and the actual infecting organism must be tested, as there is variation between different strains of the same species in the type of β lactamase produced. Although cephalosporins have been widely used in respiratory and urinary tract infections and in combination

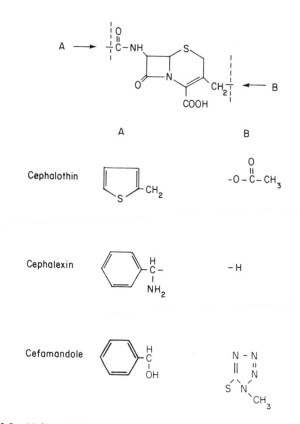

Figure XVI.9 (Adapted from Garrod, Lambert and O'Grady: *Antibiotic and Chemotherapy*, 5th Edition, by permission of Churchill Livingstone)

with other antibiotics in the treatment of severe infections, probably more experience to assess their value is needed.

Early cephalosporins

Cephalothin was one of the first cephalosporins to be used. It must be given by injection and the intramuscular route is quite painful. Cephalothin is unstable so low blood levels are produced.

Cephaloridine is rather more active than cephalothin and higher blood levels are attained. Intramuscular injection is not painful. However, it is more susceptible to staphylococcal penicillinase and may be nephrotoxic.

Cefazolin produces high concentrations in the bile and has been used in prophylaxis in surgery of the biliary tract.

Oral cephalosporins

Cephalexin is widely used and is valuable in many situations.

Cephradine is a similar compound. The relative sensitivity of these two cephalosporins to staphylococcal β lactamases has been the subject of much discussion and is perhaps not completely resolved.

β Lactamase resistant cephalosporins

Because there are many different β lactamases produced by different bacteria and because sensitivity of cephalosporins to these may vary, this has become a complex area of therapeutics. In addition there is variation in the ability of cephalosporins to penetrate the cell membrane.

Cefamandole is a useful β lactamase resistant cephalosporin because of its activity against Gram-negative bacilli, particularly *Haemophilus influenzae*.

Cefoxitin is different in structure and is a cephamycin. It is much less active than cephalosporins against Gram-positive cocci but very much more active against Gram-negative bacilli due to resistance to their β lactamases.

Cefotaxine is also relatively β lactamase resistant. In addition it has relatively low MIC's to many Gram-negative bacilli.

Broad spectrum antibiotics

Under this heading will be discussed chloramphenicol and the tetracyclines. Other antibiotics such as some of the penicillins and cephalosporins which also have a broad spectrum are considered in other sections.

Chloramphenicol

This is active against a wide range of Gram-positive and Gram-negative organisms and chlamydia. Its action is bacteriostatic. It is given by mouth and penetrates well into the cerebrospinal fluid. The usage of this antibiotic is limited due to its toxic side effects, of which bone marrow aplasia is the most important, but the incidence of this is not accurately known. A further side effect occurs in infants who may develop vomiting, refusal to feed and circulatory collapse, the 'grey syndrome'. Overgrowth of resistant organisms can occur in the alimentary tract; the organism most commonly seen being *Candida albicans*.

Chloramphenicol may be used in the treatment of *Haemophilus influenzae* meningitis, typhoid fever and occasionally in other conditions; it is particularly useful topically in the eye in the treatment of conjunctivitis.

Tetracyclines

Tetracyclines are active against Gram-positive and Gram-negative organisms, mycoplasmas, rickettsiae, and chlamydiae. Their action is bacteriostatic and they are given by mouth.

The important side effects are overgrowth in the gastro-intestinal tract of resistant organisms, particularly *Candida albicans*, and staining of the deciduous teeth. For this reason tetracycline should not be given in children under 7 years of age. In patients with impaired renal function tetracycline may produce further deterioration. The tetracyclines available are generally similar to each other in their antibacterial activity.

Tetracyclines are widely used in respiratory tract infections, particularly chronic bronchitis. Pneumococci and *Streptococcus pyogenes* may however be resistant. They are also used in the treatment of acne. As would be expected from their wide antibacterial spectrum, there are a number of other conditions particularly those due to chlamydiae and rickettsiae for which tetracyclines are useful.

Antibiotics predominantly used in the treatment of infections due to gram-positive cocci

Erythromycin

Erythromycin is active against streptococci, pneumococci, and staphylococci. It is bacteriostatic in low concentrations and bactericidal at high ones. It is acid resistant and is given orally. It is a very safe antibiotic but in the form of the estolate may give rise to liver damage. It is used for the treatment of upper respiratory tract infections particularly in children, in the treatment of diphtheria carriers and of infections due to campylobacters and *Legionella* spp.

Clindamycin

Clindamycin is active against staphylococci, pneumococci, and streptococci, and also against anaerobic bacteria. It is given by mouth. Usage of this antibiotic has declined due to the recognition of the condition, pseudomembranous colitis, which may follow its administration. This is probably due to overgrowth of toxin-producing *Clostridium difficile*. The condition may occur after administration of a number of other antibiotics although it is relatively more common with clindamycin.

The indications for the use of clindamycin include anaerobic infections due to bacteroides spp. and, because of its excellent penetration into bone, acute and chronic osteomyelitis.

Fusidic acid

Fusidic acid is active against Gram-positive bacteria and Gram-negative cocci. It is given by mouth. Side effects are mild intestinal disturbances and occasionally rashes.

It may be used for staphylococcal infections, particularly of bones and joints. Resistance develops rapidly and it may be desirable to combine it with a penicillin.

Vancomycin

Vancomycin is active against Gram-positive cocci and clostridia. It has to be given intravenously and regularly produces thrombo-phlebitis and pyrexia. Ototoxicity occurs if the serum levels are allowed to rise too high. The chief indications for its use are severe staphylococcal infections resistant to other forms of therapy.

Aminoglycosides

Gentamycin

This is the most widely used of the aminoglycosides. It is active against a wide range of Gram-negative organisms including pseudomonas, and against *Staphylococcus aureus*. It is administered parenterally usually by intramuscular injection and the chief problem of its administration is to achieve dosages which are therapeutic but non-toxic. Although complex dosage schedules have been developed, laboratory assistance is necessary. The risks of ototoxicity and nephrotoxicity are very much greater in patients with impaired renal function and in these patients monitoring of blood levels is essential. It is, however, extensively used in the treatment of serious Gram-negative infection and combined with other antibiotics in the treatment of severe infections of unknown cause.

Neomycin

This antibiotic has such severe toxic effects on the eighth nerve and the kidneys that it is only used topically on the skin or in the bladder or the bowel. The risks of absorption must be considered.

Paromomycin

This is a similar substance which is useful in the treatment of amoebic dysentery.

Kanamycin

This is less toxic than neomycin. It has a limited usage in severe Gram-negative infections but is not active against pseudomonas spp.

Tobramycin is chemically similar to kanamycin. It is used in situations where it has advantages over gentamicin. Some gentamicin resistant organisms will be tobramycin sensitive and tobramycin is more active against pseudomonas spp.

Amikacin is another kanamycin derivative. It is used at the present time for the treatment of infections resistant to other aminoglycosides.

Streptomycin

Streptomycin is active against mycobacteria and Gram-negative bacilli. It is given by intramuscular injection. Streptomycin is not now used except occasionally for the treatment of tuberculosis. Even here its use is declining due to its side effects and widespread resistance.

Peptides

The usage of all these is limited because of their toxicity.

Bacitracin

Bacitracin has a declining use in topical application to the skin.

Polymyxins

These are all active against Gram-negative bacilli including pseudomonas but excluding proteus. Two polymyxins are available for use, polymyxin B and colistin. Both can cause pain at the site of injection, paraesthesiae, numbness, weakness, dizziness, and renal damage but colistin is less painful and less toxic. The chief indication for use is pseudomonas infection. Topical preparations of polymyxins are also available. The use of polymyxin has declined with the availability of other anti-pseudomonas agents.

Sulphonamides and Trimethoprim; Other synthetic antimicrobial compounds

Sulphonamides

These are synthetic compounds and all are derived from para-amino-benzene-sulphonamide. They are active against a wide range of bacteria. There are a variety of toxic side effects including renal damage, agranulo-cytosis, and hypersensitivity reactions. A very large number of sulphonamides with different pharmacokinetics are available, including insoluble compounds used for their effect in the gut. Except in combination with trimethoprim, the usage of sulphonamides has declined very much due to the availability of other antibiotics. They are therefore not described further.

Trimethoprim

Trimethoprim is a synthetic compound which until 1979 was available for clinical use only in combination with sulphamethoxazole. This combination is called co-trimoxazole and it is used because trimethoprim is synergistic with sulphonamide. Toxic side effects occurring with its use are predominantly due to the presence of the sulphonamide. Co-trimoxazole can be used in a great variety of conditions, especially in the treatment of urinary and respiratory infections. Trimethoprim is increasingly used as a single agent, particularly in urinary infection.

Nitrofurantoin

This is given by mouth and is active against a wide range of Gram-negative bacilli. It is used almost entirely for the treatment of urinary tract infections.

Nalidixic acid

Nalidixic acid is similar in its range of activity to nitrofurantoin and is also used predominantly for the treatment of urinary tract infection.

Metronidazole

This has been used for many years to treat trichomonas infections. It has now become extremely important because of its activity against anaerobic organisms, particularly bacteroides. It is given by mouth and toxic side effects are uncommon. Its use in prophylaxis before major operations on the bowel has had a major effect in the U.K. in reducing post-operative infection rates. This is now a widely used and useful antibiotic.

Antituberculous chemotherapy

Antituberculous chemotherapy is a specialized area of therapeutics. To be satisfactory, treatment which is often prolonged must be designed so as to prevent the emergence of resistant strains of the tubercle bacillus. For this reason combinations of antibiotics are used. Therapeutic regimes introduced in the 1950s involved the usage of streptomycin, para-amino-salicylic acid (PAS), and isonicotinic acid hydrazide (INAH). Since then rifampicin has been introduced which may be used in combination with a number of other antibiotics in a variety of therapeutic regimens. Short course and intermittent chemotherapy have been fairly recent developments.

The following antituberculous antibiotics are listed merely to give the student some idea of the possibilities. The list is by no means complete.

Rifampicin

This can be given by mouth. It is very well absorbed, very active against *Mycobacterium tuberculosis* and is now extensively used. Although its toxicity is low, a great variety of side effects have been associated with its use and these vary with the dosage regime used.

Isonicotinic acid hydrazide (Isoniazid INAH)

This is an active bactericidal drug and it can be given by mouth. Some people inactivate isoniazid rapidly and others slowly. Toxic side effects are insomnia, peripheral neuritis, and psychosis, and are commoner in people who inactivate the drug slowly.

Ethambutol

This drug may cause retrobulbar neuritis and loss of vision. For this reason the dosage must be carefully controlled and patients warned of the risks.

Pyrazinamide

Pyrazinamide is hepatotoxic. However, with intermittent and short term regimes the incidence of side effects can be reduced, and it is now extensively used.

Streptomycin

Some of the properties of this antibiotic, whose usage is declining, have been given.

Para-amino-salicylic acid

This is given by mouth in large doses and regularly produces gastro-intestinal side effects. Allergic reactions and a variety of other side effects also occur. Its antituberculous activity is not great and it is only used in combination with more active antibiotics. Its usage has declined.

Antifungal antibiotics

Fungi are eucaryocytic organisms and therefore their cells are in some ways less dissimilar to human cells than are those of bacteria. For this reason the antibiotics used in the treatment of fungal infections are a different group from those used in antibacterial chemotherapy.

Polyene antibiotics

Nystatin

The name arose because this antibiotic was discovered by the New York State Department of Health. It is insoluble and is only used in local treatment of candida infections, particularly of the mouth, gut or vagina.

Amphotericin B

This drug is given intravenously for severe life-threatening fungal infections. It is usually toxic, giving rise to nausea, vomiting, thrombo-phlebitis, and renal damage. Therapy should only be commenced in severe disease.

Other anti-fungal agents

Griseofulvin

Griseofulvin is the antibiotic of choice for the treatment of dermatophyte infections. Toxic side effects are mild and uncommon. The antibiotic is given by mouth and is incorporated into the keratin of hair, skin, and nails. Treatment may need to be continued for up to 2 years.

5-Fluorocytosine

This is used in the treatment of systemic candidiasis, but results are not uniformly good and resistance to the drug may develop during treatment. Side effects include leucopenia and liver damage. Combined therapy with 5-fluorocytosine and amphotericin may be useful.

Miconazole

Miconazole is of value in the treatment of systemic candidiasis but further assessment is needed.

Antiviral antibiotics

Again because of the fundamentally different nature of viruses, a different group of agents is used for anti-viral chemotherapy than those available for the treatment of bacterial and fungal infections.

The small number and limited usefulness of the antiviral compounds available contrasts with the situation in antibacterial chemotherapy and is related to the difficulty of selectively destroying viruses which multiply within the host cell.

Interferons

These are proteins produced by cells which are infected with viruses and act by inhibiting a range of other viruses. Human leucocyte interferon is available: clinical experience with interferon is limited but indicates, however, its potential value.

Amantidine

Amantidine blocks entry of the virus into the host cell. It has been shown to be of value in influenza and to have low toxicity.

Idoxuridine

This is a thymidine analogue which inhibits thymidine synthesis. It may be used topically in herpetic infections, particularly infections of the eye.

Acyclovir

Acyclovir inhibits DNA polymerase and it is very much more active against the viral than against the mammalian enzyme. It has been used in the treatment of superficial herpes simplex infections and may also be useful in systemic disease caused by this virus.

CHAPTER XVII

Environmental Hygiene

Awareness of the role of food, milk, water, and other environmental factors in the spread of infectious diseases has done much to improve standards of hygiene in advanced countries. We expect that our water shall be pure, our food wholesome and our environment free as far as possible from dangerous poisons, noxious substances and harmful micro-organisms. Very considerable advances have been made in this direction. Water supplies are carefully protected from contamination by sewage, and regulations governing the production and distribution of food, and the destruction and control of vermin and parasites, protect us from much of the plagues, pestilences, and epidemics which were once suffered.

Other factors still operate, however, against us. For example in order to secure supplies of cheap protein it may be necessary to accept a high incidence of food poisoning organisms in products of the factory farming industry. Our rivers and beaches also are still polluted by sewage and chemical effluent. Food poisoning remains commonplace, accepted as a fact of life.

We are much dependent on a few standards, statutes and regulations governing the quality of our water, milk, and a small selection of foods. Testing specimens of these, interpreting the results and applying the regulations accordingly is vitally important.

The methods and regulations described below are those applied in the United Kingdom and are given as examples.

MILK

Almost all milk produced in the United Kingdom is now heat treated and rendered reasonably safe for consumption. Regrettably in some areas through ignorance or occasionally the mistaken idea that raw milk is preferable, untreated milk is still drunk and presents special hazards. Policies of eradication of tuberculosis and brucellosis from cattle in Britain have also much reduced the incidence of milk-borne disease but heat treatment must also be carried out. Diseases which can be milk-borne

232

include as well as tuberculosis and brucellosis, salmonellosis, campylobacter enteritis, streptococcal infections, diphtheria, dysentery, and Q
fever.

Heat Treatment

1. Pasteurization

The object of pasteurization is to kill harmful organisms in the milk
without reducing its quality as a food or impairing its taste and
appearance. The 'Holder' method requires the milk to be heated to 63°C
for 30 minutes and then cooled as rapidly as possible to below 10°C. The
'High Temperature Short Time' (HTST) method requires the
temperature of the milk to be raised to 72°C for 15 seconds and then
lowered as rapidly as possible to below 10°C. These methods will destroy
vegetative pathogens but will not of course kill spores. The milk is not
sterile.

2. Ultra heat treatment (UHT)

Milk is heated in a flow system to 132.2°C for not less than 1 second and
immediately sealed in sterile containers. Such milk yields a very low
residual count but all spores may not be killed.

3. Sterilization

In spite of its name this process in practice is not sterilization and spores
are not all killed. It is required that the milk be heated to a temperature
of above 100°C and be held at the temperature achieved for a time
sufficient to allow it to pass the 'Turbidity Test' (see below). An example
of the temperature and time normally employed is 108°C for 45 minutes.

Tests

Statutory tests for milk in the United Kingdom are minutely defined in
statutory instruments and regulations and must be carried out to the
letter. For example the way of handling milk is defined differently for
different times of the year. No attempt is made here to give details of the
tests as described in the Statutory Instruments.

1. The methylene blue test for untreated and pasteurized milk

This is the standard official method in England and Wales for gauging the keeping quality and purity of milk. It is a substitute for a bacterial count and depends on the reduction and decolorization of the dye by the bacteria in the milk. The rate of reduction affords a measure of the degree of bacterial contamination and to be satisfactory the milk must not decolorize the dye within 30 minutes; 1 ml of methylene blue is added to 10 ml of milk in a sterile test tube, closed, mixed, and put in a water bath at 37°–38°C in the dark and decolorization noted.

The strict detail of the method must be followed absolutely and for legal purposes all details of sampling, transport, storage, and testing together with the names of all those involved and the part they played must be recorded at the time.

2. The phosphatase test for pasteurized milk

The Aschaffenburg and Mullen Phosphatase Test is the statutory test for pasteurized milk. It is based on the fact that the temperature and time conditions used in the recognized methods of pasteurization, besides destroying vegetative organisms, also inactivate the enzyme phosphatase in the milk. The presence therefore of active enzyme indicates that the milk has not been adequately heated. The enzyme liberates para-nitrophenol from disodium para-nitrophenyl phosphate giving a yellow coloration which can be read in arbitrary units against controls.

3. The colony count test for ultra heat treated milk

The milk has to satisfy a colony count test by yielding less than 10 colonies per 0.01 ml when added to yeastrel agar and incubated at 30°–37°C for 48 hours.

4. The turbidity test for sterilized milk

This is the statutory test for 'sterilized' milk which has been heated to 100°C or more for an arbitrary period designed to ensure that it passes the test. Soluble proteins are denatured during the heating process. They can be precipitated in the test by ammonium sulphate and can then be removed by filtration. To be satisfactory the filtrate when subsequently boiled should show no turbidity. The test distinguishes between 'sterilized' and pasteurized milk.

5. The detection of antibiotics in raw milk

Milk which may contain antibiotics used to treat infections of the cow such as mastitis must be withheld from sale. Tests must be carried out on milk to detect infringements of this policy which could be dangerous to those allergic to an antibiotic. The test depends on the reduction of colourless 2,3,5-triphenyltetrazolium chloride (TTC) to a red precipitate of tetrazolium formazan by *Streptococcus thermophilus* in the absence of inhibitory levels of antibiotics. Penicillin contamination can be specifically demonstrated by carrying out the test in the presence of penicillinase.

6. The brucella ring test

This test detects the presence of antibodies to *Brucella abortus* in samples of milk. Pooled milk from up to 10 cows can be tested in herd screening or the method can be used to detect evidence of infection from individual cows. The antigen used to react with antibodies in the milk consists of a standardized suspension of killed *Brucella abortus* strain 99 stained with haematoxylin. In a positive reaction the antibodies in the milk sample agglutinate with the added stained antigen and rise with the cream causing the cream layer to appear dark blue or purple, while the lower layer of milk is white or very pale blue. The intensity of colour is graded +, + +, + + + or + + + +. In a negative reaction the cream layer appears lighter in colour than the milk antigen mixture or is indistinguishable from it. In tests on goats' milk the antigen/antibody complex will be seen as a sediment at the bottom of the tube rather than rise with the cream.

Attempts should be made to culture *Brucella abortus* from positive milks but of course the detection of antibodies does not necessarily mean the presence of viable organisms.

7. Other examinations

Milk can of course be examined directly for the presence of specific pathogenic organisms. Samples of pooled milk may be tested or the 'milk socks', rough filters through which milk passes in the milking parlour, may be used as a concentrating device and cultured for salmonellae, campylobacters or other organisms.

CREAM

Standards for cream are not defined as are those for milk. A methylene blue test carried out as soon after sampling as possible can be used to define grades of cream. Incubation is first at 20°C for 17 hours, and if the blue colour remains after this time further incubation at 37°C for 4 hours follows. Satisfactory cream has not decolorized the dye even at the end of the 4 hours incubation. Fairly satisfactory cream decolorizes the dye during the 4 hours incubation. Unsatisfactory cream decolorizes the dye during the initial 17 hours incubation and further samples should be tested and the organisms present identified.

ICE CREAM

A similar system may be used to grade ice cream. Samples should be transferred to the laboratory still frozen and handled aseptically. Ice cream is graded according to the times at which decolorization of the methylene blue occurs.

Decolorization within:	Grade
The first 17 hours	4
½–2 hours thereafter	3
2½–4 hours thereafter	2
Not decolorized in 4 hours	1

WATER

Drinking Water

In Britain a public supply of piped chlorinated drinking water is available to the vast majority of the population. Some people are dependent on wells or other private supplies. All water supplies, although carefully controlled, may be liable to pollution and contamination with micro-organisms, and contamination by sewage or faeces is particularly dangerous. Infections which can be water-borne include typhoid, dysentery, cholera, hepatitis, and poliomyelitis. Much of microbiological testing of water is directed to establishing whether there is evidence of faecal pollution and this is done by demonstrating the presence in the water of common faecal organisms. It is neither necessary nor practical to seek the rare and intermittent presence of human intestinal pathogens. General pollution with any organic matter can occur and the organisms sought as indicators of this are the coliforms. *Escherichia coli*, *Clostridium perfringens* and *Streptococcus faecalis* are in the same way used as indicators of actual faecal pollution and *Escherichia coli* is particularly useful in this respect.

236

All these organisms will survive for considerable periods in water but will not grow and multiply naturally in it. They can therefore be enumerated to give an estimate of the degree of pollution involved. *Clostridium perfringens* survives especially well and its presence in the absence of the other indicator organisms tends to indicate faecal pollution at an earlier date than when *Escherichia coli* is present as well.

Tests for the presence of coliforms and *Escherichia coli*

Membrane filtration

Most laboratories now use membrane filtration which is quick and relatively cheap. Two samples of water of 100 ml are taken and each is passed through a sterile filter membrane. The membranes are then placed on an absorbent pad saturated with enriched broth with lactose, phenol-red and an indicator and incubated for 4 hours at 30°C. One is then incubated at 37°C for 14 hours with very strict temperature control. Acid producing colonies are then counted and can be assumed to give an estimate of the total number of coliforms present. The other membrane is incubated at 44°C in the same way with very strict temperature control. At this temperature, acid-producing colonies can be assumed to be *Escherichia coli*. Confirmatory tests can be done on sub-cultures if required (Figs. XVII,1 and XVII,2).

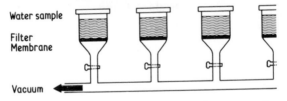

Figure XVII.1   Membrane filtration of water samples

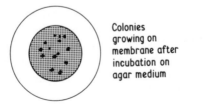

Figure XVII.2   Colonies growing on membrane

Multiple tube method

Using the same principle in the Multiple Tube Method a variety of different volumes of a suitable medium in glass tubes are inoculated with measured volumes of the water to be examined. The tubes contain inverted Durham tubes to entrap any gas produced. The production of acid and gas in any tube after incubation at 37°C indicates the presence of coliforms, and after incubation at 44°C indicates the presence of *Escherichia coli*. By comparing the numbers of positive tubes of various volumes with tables of probability, the 'Most Probable Number' of coliforms or *Escherichia coli* can be calculated (Fig. XVII,3).

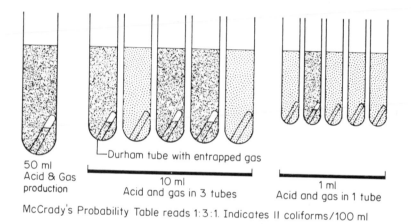

Durham tube with entrapped gas

50 ml
Acid & Gas
production

10 ml
Acid and gas in 3 tubes

1 ml
Acid and gas in 1 tube

McCrady's Probability Table reads 1:3:1. Indicates 11 coliforms/100 ml

Figure XVII.3   Multiple tube method of estimating the number of coliforms in water

Standards

Main piped supplies

Chlorinated supplies should be free from all coliforms or *Escherichia coli* at the point of entry to the system of distribution. Unchlorinated waters showing any *Escherichia coli* in 100 ml, or more than three coliforms/ 100 ml should be investigated and if the fault persists, must be chlorinated. 'User' samples taken from the distribution system, as for example from a kitchen tap, should normally be free from coliforms or *Escherichia coli* in 100 ml. Standards allow the presence, however, of very small numbers of coliforms and even *Escherichia coli* on isolated occasions.

Private small supplies

Where supplies originate from wells and springs and supply only a few people, the standards above may be unrealistic. Nevertheless contamination should be minimal and there should not be more than 10 coliforms/100 ml in the water.

Sampling

Regulations on the frequency of sampling are laid down in most countries and are becoming international, as for example in the E.E.C. They depend on the size of the undertaking. The quality of the water is primarily the responsibility of the water authority but local authorities are responsible also on behalf of the consumers. Samples are taken by trained personnel in sterile bottles containing sodium thiosulphate to neutralize any residual chlorine.

Bathing Water

Swimming pools

Pools should ideally be filtered and continually chlorinated so as to give persistent residual chlorine levels. Testing for residual chlorine is the most important test but microbiological examination can also be carried out. Samples should be taken of below-surface and surface water and residual chlorine neutralized with sodium thiosulphate. There should be no coliforms in the samples and total counts should not exceed 10/ml.

Designated bathing waters

As an example of reasonable practice E.E.C. regulations specify that it is mandatory that waters designated as suitable for bathing must not yield more than 10,000 coliforms/100 ml and that as a guideline they should not yield more than 500/100 ml. Faecal coliforms must not exceed 2,000/100 ml and should not normally exceed 100/100 ml. Having accepted that coliforms are the best indicator of pollution it is hard to understand the need for a further requirement made in the regulations that salmonellae should be absent from samples of 1,000 ml 'when their presence is suspected'.

FOOD

The microbiological examination of food is often unsatisfactory because of the difficulty or impossibility of defining either methods or standards. Examination is restricted generally to the estimation of a total count of mesophilic aerobic organisms/g and to demonstrating that there are not more than an arbitrary number of a few specific pathogens such as salmonellae, *Staphylococcus aureus* or clostridia in a sample of 1 gram of the food.

Routine Examination

The method now used when examining a food sample is to homogenize it in a diluent in a plastic bag by repeated mechanical blows between two plates. Further dilutions or subcultures can be made thereafter.

Total count

1 ml aliquots of the dilutions can be incorporated in 10–15 ml of melted agar and poured into Petri dishes. Following incubation colonies can be counted to give a 'Standard Plate Count'. Alternatively dilutions can be spread evenly on the surface of agar plates, incubated, and colonies counted to give a 'Surface Plate Count'. Economy can be practised by dropping two drops of 0.02 ml of each dilution on to a segment of an agar plate and incubating. The lowest dilution giving numerable colonies should be counted. This is a modification of a well known method described by Miles and Misra.

Examination for specific pathogens requires both enrichment and selection of the appropriate organism. Pathogenic organisms may be present in food in very small numbers and unless they are favoured in growth relative to their competitors they will not be demonstrable.

Specific organisms

Salmonellae

These are sought by methods designed to allow their isolation from specimens even when they are present in very small numbers or form a minute proportion of the total bacterial count. The sample is first grown in a lactose broth to increase the total numbers of organisms and subsequently subcultured in selective enrichment cysteine or tetrathionate broth which particularly favours the growth of salmonellae. Further subculture is on to solid media such as Brilliant Green agar designed to differentiate the colonies of salmonellae and enable them to be separated for further examination.

Staphylococcus aureus

The presence of coagulase-positive staphylococci in a food indicates that food poisoning may be caused if the food is not stored in refrigeration. It is also an indication of unsatisfactory hygiene when found in processed food. Its origin is almost certainly the skin and noses of food handlers and workers.

The dilutions used in total counts can be used to inoculate plates of various selective media which contain egg yolk. Incubation is at 37°C when *Staphylococcus aureus* appears as golden yellow shiny colonies surrounded by opalescent zones of lecithinase activity. A representative number should be checked by coagulase and DNase tests.

If greater sensitivity is required because staphylococci are present in very small numbers, as for example in suspected post-processing contamination of canned foods, enrichment techniques may be necessary by incubation in salt-meat broth.

Clostridium perfringens

This organism, which is a common environmental contaminant, spore-forming anaerobic, and resistant to heat, is usually sought and enumerated in food as a useful indicator of how satisfactory all aspects of food preparation have been, including handling, cooking, cooling, and storage.

Following dilution and homogenization a loopful of the preparation is plated out on to neomycin blood agar and incubated anaerobically for 48 hours. When very small numbers of *Clostridium perfringens* are sought, enrichment techniques can be used.

Examination in suspected food poisoning

In investigating a suspected incident of food poisoning it is important to take a careful history of those foods eaten over the previous few days and exactly when they were eaten. The symptoms are also important and vomiting, abdominal pain, diarrhoea, and pyrexia should be recorded. This information, particularly when a number of people are involved, can point clearly to the likely food and to the likely causative organism. The relative frequency of involvement of different organisms in food poisoning varies from country to country. Those which are found in Britain are listed below.

Common in Britain	Uncommon in Britain
Salmonella spp.	Escherichia coli
Staphylococcus aureus	Vibrio parahaemolyticus
Clostridium perfringens	Bacillus cereus
Campylobacter spp.	Clostridium botulinum
	Other organisms.

The main distinguishing features of bacterial food poisoning as found in Britain are summarized in Table XVII.1.

Table XVII.1

Causative organism	Onset (hours)	Duration (days)	Symptoms*	Cause
Staph. aureus	2–6	1	P,D,V	Toxin
Cl. perfringens	8–24	1–2	P,D	Infection
Cl. botulinum	24–72	1–8	D,NS	Toxin
Salmonella spp.	12–24	1–8	P,D,V,F	Infection
B. cereus serotypes 1,3,5	2–3	1–2	V	Toxin
B. cereus serotypes 2,6,8,9,10	8–15	1–2	P,D	Toxin
V. parahaemolyticus	10–15	2–5	P,D,V,F,	Infection
Campylobacter spp.	5–10 days	1–7	P,D	Infection
E. coli	18–48	1–5	P,D(V,F)	Infection

*P = Pain; D = Diarrhoea; V = Vomiting; NS = Nervous System; F = Fever.

It should be noted that some food poisoning is due to actual infection. The causative organism itself is ingested, multiplies in the bowel, elaborates its toxins there and causes the symptoms of food poisoning. In other cases the causative organism multiplies and elaborates its toxins in the food and following ingestion of this pre-formed toxin the symptoms of food poisoning result. It may not always be possible for example to demonstrate in food remains the presence of viable staphylococci when special techniques can demonstrate staphylococcal enterotoxin. Being more heat resistant than the staphylococci themselves the toxin can survive a degree of reheating or cooking which kills the organism.

The examination of suspected food when it is available follows techniques similar to those used in isolating the particular organisms from specimens of human origin and should parallel the examination of faeces and vomitus. In order to draw firm epidemiological conclusions the organisms once isolated are, where possible, typed and sub-grouped serologically or by phage-typing. The examination of food for organisms and toxins is best carried out in specially equipped Food Laboratories.

CHAPTER XVIII

Immunization

INTRODUCTION

The prevention of infectious disease by immunization has been one of the greatest contributions to human health. Prevention is always regarded as better than cure and this is especially so with regard to infectious diseases, many of which can be serious and even fatal and for the most of which there is no effective treatment. Improved hygiene, practice of the techniques of isolation and the establishment of a population protected by immunization are together dramatically reducing the incidence, morbidity and mortality of many infections, and one disease, smallpox, has been eliminated from the world.

The mechanisms of immunity are discussed in Chapter I. Artificial immunization may be Active or Passive. Active immunization depends on the introduction into the body of an antigen which stimulates the production of specific antibody, humoral or cell-mediated, to act against the appropriate infectious agent. The antigen may take the form of live organisms modified or attenuated in virulence, dead organisms or antigenic products or toxins of the organisms. Toxins are modified in practice to produce toxoids which retain antigenicity but not toxicity. When live organisms are used, a single stimulus may be sufficient to induce a good level of antibody production, although this is not always so as for example in poliomyelitis. Otherwise a good antibody level depends on a regime of initial stimulus followed 4–6 weeks later by a secondary stimulus and a third stimulus some months after that. Further 'booster' doses may be desirable at periods of years to maintain good protection against some diseases. Active immunization is the method of choice but it has the disadvantage of not providing any immediate protection against infection in the first 7–10 days after the initial stimulus and only a limited protection unless the whole schedule is completed (Fig. XVIII,1).

Passive immunization consists of providing the body with immediate protective levels of antibody by injecting ready-made antibodies produced in a human or animal in response to the appropriate antigen.

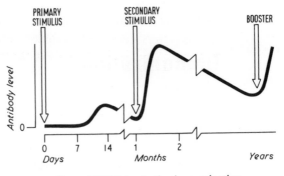

Figure XVIII.1   Active immunization

This has the advantage of giving immediate protection which active immunization cannot do. However, protection is brief as the foreign antibody gamma-globulins are soon inactivated and broken down. Specific gamma-globulins of human origin are most effective and are less quickly destroyed. Pooled human gamma-globulin is also a useful source of protection (Fig. XVIII,2).

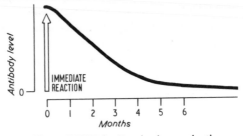

Figure XVIII.2   Passive immunization

ACTIVE IMMUNIZATION

This may best be considered as divided into:
    a) protection in childhood;
    b) protection of adults and those exposed to special hazards;
    c) protection of travellers abroad.

Immunization in childhood

Infections which are serious and preventable include diphtheria, pertussis, poliomyelitis, and tetanus. Campaigns of immunization in past years succeeded in reducing diphtheria and poliomyelitis in Britain, for example, to negligible levels and in greatly reducing the incidence, morbidity, and mortality of whooping cough. Tetanus, which is a sporadic non-epidemic disease, has become rare and much more easily treatable.

The very success of these immunization campaigns, however, has militated against continued efforts to secure high acceptance rates of immunization today in the face of what appears to the uninformed a minimal risk. In some areas acceptance rates particularly among less well educated and informed social classes are below 50%. The early problems with pertussis vaccine (see below) are particularly responsible for this situation.

A schedule of immunization in childhood is as follows.

Age		*Immunization*	
3 months	1st	Diphtheria	Triple vaccine 0.5 ml
5 months	2nd	Tetanus	I.M. or deep subcutaneous
		Pertussis	
9 months	3rd	and Oral Poliomyelitis	
1½–2 years		Measles vaccine	
4–5 years		Diphtheria	Booster on entering school
		Tetanus	or nursery school
		and Oral Poliomyelitis	
11–13 years		Rubella vaccine (girls)	
		Tuberculin testing and BCG if required	
16–18 years		Tetanus and Oral Poliomyelitis	on leaving school

Diphtheria

It is vitally necessary to provide antibody against the toxin of *Coryne-bacterium diphtheriae*. This is achieved by using formol toxoid absorbed on to aluminium phosphate. The vaccine is usually used in combination with tetanus and pertussis vaccines as 'Triple Vaccine' or with tetanus alone in the immunization of infants. Adults and children over 10 years must on no account be immunized against diphtheria, unless they are shown *not* to have acquired immunity by demonstrating a positive Schick Test. This test should be carried out with extreme care. An intradermal injection of 0.1 ml of diluted diphtheria toxin is made in one forearm and a similar inactivated control is injected in the other arm. A positive reaction shows redness in the test alone lasting up to 4–5 days, ending in pigmentation and desquamation before it fades. Diphtheria vaccine must not be given to Schick-negative individuals as the reaction may be severe. Schick-positive adults, or children over 10 years, can be immunized if necessary using Diphtheria Vaccine TAF, a suspension of floccules prepared from diphtheria formol-toxoid. The measurement of diphtheria antitoxin levels in serum by demonstrating a level of protection against the cytopathic effect of diphtheria toxin on tissue culture cells is now available.

Tetanus

The most important factor in tetanus is the very powerful neurotropic exotoxin elaborated by the organism. The object of immunization is to stimulate the production of antibody against this toxin. A formol toxoid is used and may be adsorbed on a mineral carrier such as aluminium hydroxide to improve antigenicity. In childhood it is generally given in combination with diphtheria and pertussis vaccines. Everyone should be immunized against tetanus so that following wounds and injuries their immunity need only be boosted. A further dose of tetanus toxoid is given if the patient has not received a dose within 1 year and the injury is major or penetrating, contaminated or involving destruction of tissue. If the injury is slight and superficial and clean, a boosting dose need only be given if there has been no immunization in the previous 5 years. Too many frequent booster doses may cause hypersensitivity reactions. If an injured patient has no immunity it may be necessary to give anti-tetanus immunoglobulin and a full course of active immunization.

Pertussis

Whooping cough can be one of the most serious infections of infancy and childhood, with serious morbidity and significant mortality in the early months of life. Pertussis vaccine is generally given as part of 'Triple Vaccine' together with diphtheria and tetanus, but is available separately as Pertussis Vaccine (Per/Vac) and can be given as 0.5 ml by intramuscular or deep subcutaneous injection. It consists of a preparation of killed *Bordetella pertussis* organisms.

Pertussis vaccine may give rise to some side effects usually confined to local reactions with low grade pyrexia and restlessness. The association of pertussis vaccination with convulsions and encephalopathy is highly controversial. It arose 20 years ago and although not specifically proven was sufficiently believed to do great damage to the reputation of the vaccine.

Not only were children not immunized against pertussis, but the uptake of other immunization in childhood was adversely affected as well. The vaccine used in 1960 was not that used today. The contra-indications to pertussis vaccination, it is hoped, are much better understood and accepted today. The first dose of the vaccine is now recommended at 3 months instead of 6 months so that the most vulnerable children are protected, and yet the bad reputation remains. The Department of Health in England and Wales in 1981 reviewed the contra-indications to pertussis vacine. The vaccine is absolutely contra-indicated where there is:

a) a history of any severe local or general reaction (including neurological reaction) to a preceding dose;
b) a history of cerebral irritation or damage in the neonatal period, or of fits or convulsions.

Vaccination should be postponed if the child is suffering from any acute febrile illness, particularly respiratory, until fully recovered. Minor infections without fever or systemic upset are not regarded as a contra-indication.

Certain groups of children in whom whooping cough vaccination is not absolutely contra-indicated require special consideration as to its advisability:

a) children whose parents or siblings have a history of idiopathic epilepsy;
b) children with developmental delay thought to be due to a neurological defect;
c) children with neurological disease.

The very important point is made that while the risk of vaccination may be higher than in normal children the effects of whooping cough may also be more severe. It is absolutely essential that even when pertussis vaccine is contra-indicated an infant should still be considered for immunization against diphtheria and tetanus.

Poliomyelitis

Sabine.

There are three major strains of the virus of poliomyelitis antigenically distinct and it is necessary to induce the production of antibodies to all three strains. Poliomyelitis vaccine may be inactivated and given by subcutaneous or intramuscular injection in a course of three doses, or it may be live attenuated vaccine given orally again in a course of three doses. In either case the vaccine contains all three strains of virus. The inactivated vaccine is only used to immunize those for whom the oral vaccine is contra-indicated, such as those with chronic diarrhoea or hypogammaglobulinaemia. Although the oral vaccine is a live vaccine it must be given on three occasions as the different strains in it may interfere one with another in the gut and prevent the proper development of immunity.

Side effects with oral poliovaccine are rare but very occasionally the virus may gain neurovirulence in the gut and excreted organisms may very rarely cause vaccine virus infection in close contacts. For this reason the parents of babies being immunized may be offered coincidental vaccination especially if they are themselves young.

Measles

Although it is a very common childhood fever, measles can be serious and very occasionally lead to complications such as encephalitis. For these reasons vaccination against measles is recommended in the second year of life. A live attenuated measles virus is used, 0.5 ml by a single subcutaneous or intramuscular injection. Very good and lasting immunity is achieved. There are frequent mild side effects of rash and pyrexia simulating a mild measles infection. Encephalitis, very rare in natural measles, is very much rarer following vaccination. Measles vaccination should be deferred until the age of 2–3 years in epileptic children or those with a history of convulsions, and the reaction may be modified by giving normal immunoglobulin at the time of vaccination.

Rubella

Rubella is a very mild childhood fever, often undiagnosed, and there is no indication for immunization to protect children against it. Rubella infection, however, of a pregnant woman, especially if it occurs in the first 3 or 4 months, can severely damage the foetus. For this reason it is important that all girls be immunized before reaching child-bearing age and this is advised at 11–13 years of age. Immunized girls must not be pregnant at the time and must not become pregnant for at least 3 months. The chance of damage to a foetus from the vaccine is very small but cannot be risked. The vaccine is a live attenuated virus given in a 0.5 ml dose subcutaneously or intramuscularly.

Tuberculosis

It is accepted that anyone at risk of infection with *M. tuberculosis* should be offered immunization against the disease. It is the practice in the UK to carry out tuberculin testing of children aged 11-13 years. This is carried out using 'tuberculin', an extract of *M. tuberculosis* which is introduced into the skin of the forearm. The Heaf test employs a multiple puncture technique while the Mantoux test requires intradermal injection using a fine needle. Reaction by induration and reddening is a 'POSITIVE' result and such a person is regarded as having achieved a state of hypersensitivity to *M. tuberculosis* which is protective against the effects of subsequent infection. Those giving a 'NEGATIVE' reaction are vaccinated using a live attenuated strain of *M. tuberculosis*, the 'Bacille Calmette Guérin' or BCG. This is introduced intracutaneously exactly above the insertion of the deltoid muscle giving rise to a small ulcer which heals after 2-3 months. Subsequent tuberculin testing if carried out should show a conversion to a positive reaction. Patients should not be given BCG unless tuberculin negative. There is no evidence that those who have once been tuberculin positive but who subsequently revert to a tuberculin negative state are any more susceptible to infection than those who remain positive. In some countries tuberculin negative individuals are not given BCG, but people who convert to become tuberculin positive are treated, usually with isoniazid.

The improvement in living conditions and the health of many communities has in the last decades meant that to many there is now little risk of infection with *M. tuberculosis* and the need for immunization is questionable. Such groups which are identified as specially at risk should be immunized, and where tuberculosis is rife, BCG immunization should be given to neonates without delay.

Immunization in Adult Life

Immunization in adult life will depend to a considerable extent on what particular risks are likely to be run by an individual. It is worthwhile to try to confer immunity to a number of infectious diseases when the adult has not been immunized in childhood.

Rubella

All women of child-bearing age should be tested for the presence of natural acquired antibodies or antibodies acquired after artificial active immunization with rubella vaccine. Those adjudged to be susceptible should be offered rubella vaccination on the strict understanding that they are not pregnant and will not become pregnant for at least 3 months following vaccination. It is usual to test women in pregnancy in antenatal clinics and to vaccinate the susceptible women immediately after the birth of the child. Hospital staff and others at special risk are also offered immunization if unprotected so as to avoid their infecting patients who are of low resistance or immunologically compromised.

Poliomyelitis

Any adult not previously immunized should be offered a full course of oral vaccine with 6–8 weeks between the first and second dose and 4–6 months between the second and third. A booster dose should be given if the patient is at risk as a contact thereafter.

Tetanus

All adults, particularly those in contact with soil, road dirt or in any hazardous occupation in which they are liable to injury, should be immunized against tetanus in the following schedule. The first dose should be followed by a second after 6–8 weeks and a third after a further 6 months. Subsequent booster doses need not be more often than every 10 years or in case of injury.

Influenza

The antigenic variations of influenza make it essential that the vaccine offered is constantly updated to contain those antigens adjudged most likely to become prevalent in the community, and monitoring of strains of influenza continues on a world-wide basis to detect variations and trends.

The vaccine consists of purified and inactivated virus products and is usually given as a single dose intramuscularly at the start of the winter. It is offered to groups of people in whom the infection could prove particularly serious. These include the old, particularly those suffering from chronic bronchitis, heart disease or nephritis, or others with reduced resistance and vitality. It may also be offered to workers at special risk of infection or to any key worker of particular importance to the community.

Immunization of Those Exposed to Special Hazards

Protection of workers in infectious diseases wards, ambulancemen, staff of microbiology laboratories and post mortem rooms, and those similarly at risk requires immunization against the diseases considered above. Reinforcement may be more frequent, for example poliomyelitis vaccine should be given every 3 years. Immunization against diseases such as typhoid and anthrax may be given if appropriate.

Immunization of Travellers Abroad

It is no longer necessary on medical grounds to vaccinate against smallpox in any part of the world, although a handful of countries may still demand a certificate of vaccination. The need for immunization against other serious infections varies depending on which countries are to be visited or passed through however briefly. Details of the specific requirements are published by the Departments of Health or may be available from embassies and consulates. Immunization should not be left to the last minute but planned sensibly in advance.

Yellow fever

The vaccine consists of a live attenuated virus, and a single dose will give protection from about 10 days after vaccination for a period of up to 10 years. It is usually accepted that infants under 9 months should not be vaccinated. An international certificate of vaccination will be issued by the vaccination centre.

Cholera

A vaccine is available in the form of killed cholera vibrios. Immunization does offer some protection but it is not complete and is of short duration. Two doses should be given with an interval of 4–6 weeks and a booster dose should be given after 6 months if exposure is continuing. An international certificate of vaccination is issued.

Typhoid and paratyphoid

It may be considered advisable to seek some protection at least against typhoid and a vaccine is available consisting of killed *Salmonella typhi*. Two doses are given with an interval of 4–6 weeks. Protection is not complete but the severity of the infection and its mortality are significantly reduced.

Poliomyelitis

Immunization is of course advisable for children and adults in any case but is particularly so if proceeding abroad. An immunized person should receive a boosting dose if going to warm countries.

Rabies

Immunization against rabies is confined to those at risk because of their occupation or in special circumstances following exposure. Immunization is usually given following scratching or biting by an animal which is suspected of being rabid.

A course of five injections of killed rabies vaccine, prepared from virus grown on human diploid cells, is begun, together with passive immunization by specific immunoglobulin when the risk is judged to be particularly serious. Immediate first aid must also be carried out to any scratch or wound. It is important that the suspect animal be caught and examined if possible.

PASSIVE IMMUNIZATION

This is achieved by direct inoculation of the patient with pre-formed antibodies. These have been produced in a person or animal in response to the appropriate antigen. Specific antisera containing antibodies against some single infectious agents are available and pooled human immunoglobulin can be used in other cases.

Normal Human Immunoglobulin

Rubella

If a susceptible woman in the first 3 months of pregnancy is in contact with rubella, an intramuscular injection of 750 mg of immunoglobulin may be of value in preventing damage to the foetus. It must be given as soon as possible after the contact.

Infectious hepatitis

Patients at particular risk who are known to have been in contact with infectious hepatitis may be given immunoglobulin to prevent or modify the infection. Young children should be given 250 mg and adults and children of more than 10 years 500 mg. Travellers to countries with poor hygiene where the disease is endemic can be afforded some protection for a few months. The injection should be given just before departure.

Measles

Susceptible debilitated children or those with reduced resistance should receive some protection if exposed to infection. It may be thought desirable not to prevent entirely the threatened attack but merely to attenuate it. The appropriate dose of normal human immunoglobulin is as follows:

Prevention:	<1 year	250 mg
	1–2 years	500 mg
	3 years and over	750 mg
Attenuation:		250 mg

Specific Immunoglobulins

These are generally very expensive and in short supply. They should only be given when patients are considered to be at genuine risk if they should contact the particular disease either because they are very young or leukaemic or have reduced immunocompetence. Those available are as follows.

Anti-varicella-zoster immunoglobulin

This should be given following close contact with chickenpox or zoster.

Prevention	<1 year	500 mg
	1–6 years	1.0 g
	7 years and over	1.5 g

Normal human immunoglobulin can be used when specific immunoglobulin is not available to attenuate an attack.

Anti-mumps immunoglobulin

This is given to close contacts with mumps.

Prevention:	<1 year	500 mg
	1–6 years	1.0 g
	7 years and over	1.5 g

750 mg–1500 mg of normal immunoglobulin can be used when specific immunoglobulin is not available.

Anti-hepatitis B immunoglobulin

This should only be given in carefully controlled circumstances when a clearly defined accident has taken place involving the inoculation of the patient with known positive material. Before it is given the recipient must be known to be negative for carriage of HB_S antigen or HB_S antibody. A vaccine of HB_SAg has been developed to allow active immunization and is now available.

The use of antisera in the treatment or prevention of Botulism, Diphtheria, Tetanus, and Rabies is described in the sections on these diseases.

CHAPTER XIX

Laboratory Methods Used in Diagnosis

The diagnosis of infectious disease is made either directly by demonstrating the presence of the infecting organism in the lesion or indirectly by measuring the response of the infected host to the presence of the organism.

Demonstration of the presence of the organism is usually carried out by culturing it from specimens taken from the lesion but much less commonly it may be done by microscopy of specially stained tissue sections or smears or by the demonstration of the presence of an antigen or product of the micro-organism in body fluids or tissue.

The response of the host is measured by looking for high or rising titres of antibodies or, again less commonly, by demonstrating a cellular response to a recognized antigen.

DEMONSTRATION OF THE PRESENCE OF THE ORGANISM

Specimens for examination

Demonstration of the presence of the organism is the most common way of making a diagnosis particularly in bacterial infections. An appropriate specimen is taken; this may be sputum, urine, pus, blood, faeces, cerebrospinal fluid, or tissue. The value of the results obtained in a diagnostic laboratory is highly dependent on the quality of the specimen received. In the case of urine, the importance of the methods of collection and transport have already been stressed. Pus is a very useful specimen and should be sent in a sterile universal container. The temptation to send a swab of the pus should be resisted. The swab is liable to dry out resulting in the death of some bacteria and it cannot be used to demonstrate characteristic bacterial products by techniques such as gas–liquid chromatography. Blood for culture is taken aseptically into liquid culture media. The avoidance of contamination is important, as it is often difficult to distinguish contaminants from opportunistic pathogens. The skin and the cap of the blood culture bottle must be carefully cleaned, and skill in venepuncture is most important. In the case of cerebrospinal fluid, careful aseptic techniques must be practised both to prevent the introduction of organisms into the body and to avoid contamination of the specimen. A blood contaminated specimen is also undesirable as it complicates the interpretation of the white cell counts. Faecal specimens present no particular problems but in the diagnosis of amoebic dysentery a freshly passed specimen, brought directly to the laboratory, is needed to demonstrate the motile organisms. Biopsy material is valuable and difficult to repeat and every care should be taken to ensure that it is handled correctly.

Viruses are less commonly cultured than bacteria, but if this is to be done it must be remembered that the techniques used are more expensive and time-consuming and that it is particularly important that suitable specimens are sent. Most specimens are transported in viral transport medium and must be kept cold either in ice or in solid carbon dioxide until processed.

Many laboratories issue a laboratory guide which includes information about types of specimens required for particular investigations. Once the specimen is received in the laboratory it is examined microscopically and by culture.

Microscopy

In the case of most specimens received in the laboratory for bacterial examination this is done by Gram-staining a smear of the specimen. This may give a strong indication of the type of organism present and in the case of CSF it may be possible to identify reasonably definitely the causative organism.

The Ziehl–Neelsen stain may be used for the demonstration of mycobacteria. The presence of acid and alcohol fast bacilli must be interpreted with caution in some specimens but in the case of sputum such an appearance is nearly always diagnostic of tuberculosis. Fluorescent staining of tubercle bacilli is used to facilitate the reading of smears.

The Romanowsky stains are used to demonstrate cellular appearances and some parasites, particularly malaria in blood films. These stains are formed by the interaction of eosin and methylene blue and they stain the chromatin of malaria and other parasites reddish purple. There are a number of Romanowsky stains. Leishman's stain is often used for protozoa in blood and Giemsa's stain may also be used for this and for staining spirochaetes.

Very occasionally more specific staining techniques are carried out. Albert's stain is used to demonstrate the volutin granules in *Corynebacterium diphtheriae* and the presence of spores may be demonstrated using special spore stains.

Microscopy of unstained specimens is used in diagnostic laboratories mainly in three types of situation. The commonest one is the examination of urine for the presence of white blood cells and casts, the others are the use of dark-ground microscopy to demonstrate the morphology of spirochaetes in the diagnosis of syphilis and the examination of faeces for the presence of parasites and their ova.

In the diagnosis of viral infections, light microscopy may be used to demonstrate inclusion bodies. This is also commonly done for chlamydial eye infections. Electron microscopy of clinical material is also useful and is sometimes used to demonstrate rotaviruses with their characteristic morphology in the faeces of infants.

Immunofluorescent staining of tissues and other specimens using fluorescent labelled antibodies has been little used in diagnostic work. The attempts that have been made have generally failed due to lack of specificity in the antisera used and sharing of antigens between different micro-organisms, although some success has been achieved in the rapid diagnosis of viral infections.

Cultural Methods

Culture of bacteria and fungi

Liquid and solid culture media may be used. Liquid media are of less value in diagnostic work as they cannot be used to separate mixtures of organisms. They are used mainly in the diagnosis of septicaemia, when the blood will almost always only contain one type of organism. Solid media generally have an agar base, although inspissated serum and egg media are also used. Loeffler's serum slopes are valuable in the diagnosis of diphtheria, and egg-containing media such as Dorset's egg and Loewenstein–Jensen medium in the diagnosis of tuberculosis. The agar media commonly used are valuable as they enable mixtures of organisms to be separated and a presumptive identification of many bacteria can be made on their colonial appearance.

Both liquid and solid media may be totally synthetic and chemically defined but the media used in diagnostic work are almost always based on aqueous extracts of meat and peptone. These media may be enriched by the addition of blood, heated blood or other substances without which many human pathogens cannot be cultured. Selective, enrichment, and indicator media may be used (Chapter I). Hundreds of different types of media are available and may be used for particular purposes.

Culture of viruses

Viruses will multiply only in living cells, as will some highly parasitic bacteria, the chlamydiae and rickettsiae. Cells are usually provided as tissue cultures. These are really cell cultures which may be derived from normal or malignant cells. The tissue cultures derived from normal cells will divide only for a few generations, but cell lines such as HeLa cells derived from carcinomas will divide indefinitely. A large number of different cell lines may be used for different viruses.

The other methods available for culturing viruses make use of fertile hens' eggs and whole animals. Inoculation of fertile hens' eggs may be on to the chorio-allantoic membrane or into the amniotic, allantoic or yolk sacs. Eggs are not now often used, but the appearance of pox and herpes viruses on the chorio-allantois is characteristic. Whole animals are still necessary very occasionally. Intracerebral inoculation of suckling mice in the isolation of Coxsackie A viruses is an example.

Growth of the virus in tissue culture may be detected by its cytopathic effect. This is a change in cell appearance which may be rounding, shrinking or ballooning (Fig. XIX,1). Multi-nucleated giant cells may be produced. In the case of viruses which multiply without producing a visible cytopathic effect, their presence may be detected in a number of ways. Haemagglutinating virus may be detected by the addition of erythrocytes which adhere to infected cells; fluorescent labelled antibody may be used or the cells already infected may be demonstrated to be

Monolayer of
normal cells

Monolayer showing
cytopathic effect

Figure XIX.1   One type of viral cytopathic effect

immune to further infection with other viruses which produce a demonstrable cytopathic effect (interference).

Identification of cultured bacteria and fungi

Once organisms have been cultured, identification is often necessary. The level to which this needs to be carried is variable. For example, in the case of a Gram-negative bacillus isolated from urine in significant numbers, there may be little reason from the point of view of the individual patient for a detailed identification, although it is necessary to exclude salmonella infection. However, if there is any doubt that an outbreak of nosocomial infection may be occurring, detailed identification and typing may be necessary for epidemiological purposes. At the other extreme a corynebacterium isolated from a throat swab, if it shows any of the characteristics of *C. diphtheriae*, must be fully identified and in particular toxin production by the organism must be looked for.

The identification of organisms is, therefore, carried out either to enable an assessment of their pathogenicity to be made or for epidemiological purposes.

Identification of bacteria may be carried out using biochemical tests. These tests include those designed to show which carbohydrates are utilized and whether this is aerobic or anaerobic.

Fermentation tests, for example, are regularly used to determine which carbohydrates are split with the production of acid and the pH change shown by an indicator colour range. Fermentation of lactose, glucose, maltose, sucrose, and many other compounds is often looked for. To distinguish between aerobic and anaerobic breakdown special anaerobic media are available.

The presence of breakdown products and the ability to utilize particular substrates for growth are also identification methods, but are less common. The methyl-red test and Voges–Proskauer test demonstrate a low pH (below 4.5) and the production of acetyl methyl carbinol. These tests are used in the identification of enterobacteria. Citrate utilization as the sole carbon and energy source is an example of the utilization of a particular substrate and again is valuable in the identification of enterobacteria.

Once the bacteria have been identified, serological tests are available to provide a more specific identification, as in the salmonellae. Serological tests may also be used to type bacteria and this may be useful to identify particular pathogenic strains or for epidemiological purposes.

Methods of isolating and identifying fungi are very similar to those described for bacteria.

Identification of viruses

The final viral identification is carried out by demonstration of neutralization of the cytopathic effect, of haemadsorption or of interference by specific antisera.

Diagnosis by demonstration of microbial antigens

The rapid diagnosis of bacterial infections by detection of specific bacterial antigens is used particularly in the examination of fluids which are normally sterile. Its chief value is in the diagnosis of bacterial meningitis which is usually due to one of a small number of organisms. The bacterial antigen may be detected by a number of serological techniques and counter-immunoelectrophoresis is often used.

In the diagnosis of viral infections, the most important antigens demonstrated are those of hepatitis B virus present in the blood of the infected individual.

Detection of microbial products

A number of attempts have been made to introduce automated and rapid diagnostic procedures into clinical microbiology. For example, one of these, gas–liquid chromatography, is used to detect infection with organisms such as anaerobes or mycobacteria. The use of this and other techniques to produce a rapid diagnosis is likely to increase in the future.

DEMONSTRATION OF INFECTION USING THE PATIENT'S IMMUNE RESPONSE

The production of antibodies or of a cellular immune response to an infecting organism may be used in the diagnosis of many infections. The immunological response is so specific that in many instances the pathogen may be precisely identified.

Serological methods

Serological methods are used in two main ways in diagnostic microbiology. As described previously, an unknown organism isolated from a patient may be identified by the demonstration of specific antigens on its surface, using known antisera. Using known organisms, antibodies present in patients' serum may be demonstrated and their presence used to diagnose previous or current infection. The diagnosis of infection usually involves the demonstration of a rising titre of antibodies to the infecting organism, although a single high level may be diagnostic of a particular infection. The presence of the antibodies may be demonstrated by a variety of techniques. These include direct agglutination of the infecting organism by the patient's serum, precipitin tests, complement fixation, fluorescent antibody labelling, radio-immuno-assay, Elisa techniques and many others. The techniques used may be refined by detecting different immunoglobulin classes. The demonstration of IgM antibody indicating recent infection is of particular importance in considering the diagnosis of brucellosis and of rubella, particularly in pregnancy.

Although many new serological techniques have been introduced, the ones commonly used are agglutination, precipitation and complement fixation. A variety of techniques are used in the diagnosis of syphilis and brucellosis and are discussed with these diseases.

Diseases diagnosed by serological tests include those in which isolation of the organism is impossible, difficult or time-consuming. They include most viral infections, many parasitic diseases, brucellosis, syphilis, Legionnaire's disease and many others.

Cellular immune responses

These are used in the diagnosis of infections in which the immunological response is the development of delayed hypersensitivity. The most commonly used test is the Heaf test, which is the intradermal inoculation of the Purified Protein Derivative of *M. tuberculosis*. A positive result is indicated by an area of reddening and induration surrounding the injection site and indicates previous contact with the antigen or a closely related one. Similar tests may be used in the diagnosis of leprosy, brucellosis, and lymphogranuloma venereum.

EXAMPLES OF METHODS OF INVESTIGATION OF SPECIMENS COMMONLY EXAMINED IN A DIAGNOSTIC LABORATORY

It should be noted that the technical details given here are designed to indicate to the medical student the main outline of the laboratory techniques used. An individual wishing to carry out these tests should consult more detailed technical publications.

Urine

1) Receive refrigerated or in a borate bottle.

2) Examine under low power of microscope for white blood cells, red blood cells and casts.

3) Inoculate a MacConkey agar plate using a standard loop.

4) Examine culture after overnight incubation. If more than 10^5 organisms/ml are present, determine the sensitivity to antibiotics commonly used in urinary tract infection, e.g. ampicillin, trimethroprim with and without sulphonamide, nalidixic acid, and nitrofurantoin.

5) Report indicating clearly whether infection is present or not and if it is, the antibiotic sensitivity of the infecting organism.

Faeces

1) Inoculate on to selenite medium for salmonellas, deoxycholate media for shigellas, MacConkey agar for enteropathogenic *E. coli* (if patient is under 3 years of age), to Thayer–Martin media for campylobacters (incubate at 43°C), and TCBS agar for vibrios.

Inoculate faeces to Robertson's cooked meat medium, steam for 30 minutes and subculture to blood agar aerobically for *B. cereus* and to blood agar anaerobically for *Clostridium perfringens*.

2) Examine deoxycholate medium for the pale colonies of non-lactose fermenters, subculture selenite broth to deoxycholate medium and examine after overnight incubation in the same way. If non-lactose fermenters are present, exclude *Proteus* spp. by inoculation to a urea slope. If urea is split, discard. If urea is not split, identify by biochemical tests followed by slide and tube agglutination reactions for detailed identification.

Take five coliform colonies from the MacConkey plate and carry out a slide agglutination reaction using polyvalent *E. coli* antisera. If negative, discard. If positive, look for agglutination with the individual constituents of the pool and confirm using a tube agglutination technique and a boiled suspension of *E. coli* to preserve to O antigen.

Confirm identity as *E. coli* using routine biochemical tests.

Examine Thayer Martin and TCBS media after 48 hours incubation for campylobacters and vibrios, and blood agar aerobically for *B. cereus* and anaerobically for heat-resistant *Cl. perfringens*.

3) Even if pathogens are isolated, many intestinal infections do not normally require antibiotic therapy. It is usual to determine the sensitivity of the infecting organism as a safeguard against the unlikely event of the development of very severe or generalized disease.

4) If the patient has been to an area where cholera and typhoid are endemic, then these are examined for. Typhoid will be isolated by the scheme described above for other salmonellas. Cholera will be isolated on TCBS media and identified using specific antisera.

5) If no pathogens are isolated, the faeces may be examined for viruses. Electron microscopy may demonstrate rotaviruses, coronaviruses and adenoviruses.

6) Parasites may be examined for in the following way:

  a) a fresh stool for the active trophozoites of *Entamoeba histolytica*;
  b) formol ether concentration can be used to demonstrate the characteristic ova of helminths and the cysts of *Entamoeba hystolytica*. In this technique the faeces are shaken with formol ether and the ova are concentrated in the surface layer and can be demonstrated microscopically. *Enterobius vermicularis* (threadworm or pinworm) ova are demonstrated by examination of a piece of transparent adhesive tape which is stuck to the perianal skin and then laid flat on a microscope slide.

Blood culture

1) The skin is cleaned with 70% ethyl alcohol or with isopropyl alcohol. Blood is taken aseptically. The cap of the blood culture bottle is cleaned with alcohol and 5–10 ml of blood is added to the liquid medium. Glucose broth is one of a variety of media which may be used and incubation may be carried out in air or with added CO_2. If anaerobes are suspected, thioglycollate broth is useful.

2) Examine the cultures after overnight incubation by naked eye, Gram-staining and subculture. Thereafter, examine the bottles at 3, 5, and 10 days and then discard unless brucellosis is suspected, when incubation for 3 weeks is necessary.

3) Any positive blood cultures are immediately reported to the ward and the antibiotic sensitivity delivered as rapidly as possible.

Wound swabs and pus

1) Gram-stain the specimen and record the presence of pus cells and organisms.

2) Inoculate the specimen on to blood agar and MacConkey agar for aerobic incubation and on to blood agar for anaerobic incubation.

3) Examine the plates at 24 hours and if necessary at 48 and 72 hours. The organisms looked for include staphylococci, streptococci, Gram-negative bacilli, clostridia and bacteroides. Identify them by the colonial appearance, Gram stain, ability to grow aerobically and anaerobically and biochemical reactions. Determine the antibiotic sensitivity of all isolates.

Sputum

1) Examine the specimen macroscopically and microscopically to determine whether sputum or saliva has been sent. If only saliva is present, discard the specimen and request a repeat. If sputum is available, Gram-stain a purulent area and culture on blood and heated blood agar. Examine the cultures particularly for *Haemophilus influenzae* and *Streptococcus pneumoniae*. They are distinguished by their colonial appearance and morphology on Gram-staining. *Haemophilus influenzae* is also identified by its requirement for X & V factors and *Streptococcus pneumoniae* is distinguished from *Streptococcus viridans* by its sensitivity to optochin. Many other organisms may be isolated from sputum, including Gram-negative bacilli. The status of these organisms as pathogens is difficult to define.

Cerebrospinal fluid

The specimen is taken using aseptic technique and is sent to the laboratory in a plain bottle.

1) Examine by naked eye.

2) Determine the protein and glucose levels.

3) Carry out a white and red cell count.

4) Centrifuge and Gram-stain the centrifuged deposit. Identify the white cells present as polymorphonuclear leucocytes or lymphocytes and look for the presence of bacteria.

5) Inoculate the deposit on to blood agar and heated blood agar. Carry out direct sensitivity tests to penicillin, sulphonamide, chloramphenicol, and ampicillin.

6) Examine for the presence of bacterial antigens in the CSF by immuno-electrophoresis or latex agglutination tests.

7) Incubate plates for 24 and if necessary 48 hours in the presence of $5-10\%$ CO_2. Examine for any growth. The organisms commonly isolated

include *Haemophilus influenzae*, pneumococci, meningococci, and, in neonates, coliforms. Identify by Gram-staining and other properties including biochemical reactions.

8) In the presence of a lymphocytosis, examine for tubercle bacilli by staining by the Ziehl-Neelsen method and by culture. Viral infections are much more common and may be examined for by tissue culture of the CSF.

Urethral discharge

1) Gram-stain the discharge. Look for the presence of Gram-negative intracellular diplococci. Their presence in the male is diagnostic of gonorrhoea.

2) Culture on heated blood agar in the presence of 5–10% CO_2 and examine after 24 and 48 hours incubation for Gram-negative diplococci. Determine penicillin sensitivity and look for β lactamase production. Confirm identity by biochemical reactions, fluorescent antibody tests or co-agglutination.

3) In cases of non-gonococcal urethritis, look for chlamydia by tissue culture techniques.

High vaginal swabs

1) Examine pus directly in warm saline for motile *Trichomonas vaginalis*.

2) Gram-stain and examine for Gram-negative diplococci and for *Candida albicans*. Look for penetration of epithelial cells by the pseudo-hyphae of candida indicating active infection.

3) Culture on heated blood agar, incubate in 10% carbon dioxide and examine at 24 and 48 hours for *Neisseria gonorrhoeae*. Also culture on Sabouraud's agar and examine for *Candida albicans*. Following childbirth, abortion, and gynaecological surgery, any high vaginal swabs should be treated as wound swabs.

Serological investigations

Syphilis

A useful combination of tests used in many laboratories is the VDRL with the TPHA and absorbed FTA tests.

a) VDRL (Venereal Disease Research Laboratory) Flocculation test

1) Inactivate serum for 30 mins at 56°C.
2) Make up antigen and use within 24 hours.
3) Mix reagents on a slide, rotate on a mechanical slide rotator. Examine for flocculation (Fig. XIX,2).

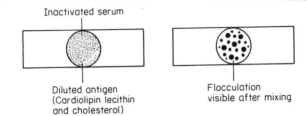

Inactivated serum

Diluted antigen
(Cardiolipin lecithin
and cholesterol)

Flocculation
visible after mixing

Figure XIX.2   VDRL (Venereal Disease Research Laboratory) Flocculation Test

This test may also be carried out in tubes and made quantitative by using serial dilutions of the serum.

b) TPHA test (Treponema pallidum haemagglutination)

1) Inactivate patient's serum at 56°C for 30 minutes.
2) Make serial dilution of patient's serum and add to turkey red blood cells with and without treponemal antigen.
3) Mix. Leave at room temperature for 1 hour.
4) Read for agglutination and record titre of sera (Fig. XIX,3).

c) FTA Abs test (Absorbed Fluorescent Treponemal Antibody)

1) Place a loopful of treponemal suspension on a slide (Nichol's strain of *Treponema pallidum* is used). Dry and fix in methanol.
2) Inactivate sera and mix with absorbing agent. This is a treated suspension of Reiter treponemes which will remove group antigens. Leave for 30 minutes.
3) Add one drop of serum absorbent mixture to the slide. Incubate at 37°C for 30 minutes in a moist chamber.
4) Rinse. Add 1 drop of fluorescent anti-human globulin. Again incubate at 37°C for 30 minutes. Rinse.
5) Examine by fluorescence microscopy. Look for fluorescing treponemes and compare with known positive and negative controls (Fig. XIX,4).

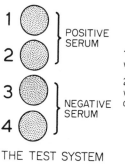

POSITIVE SERUM

1 & 3 Turkey red cells with no antigen

2 & 3 Turkey red cells with treponemal antigen

NEGATIVE SERUM

THE TEST SYSTEM

1, 3 & 4 Non-agglutinated red cells forming a 'button' at base of the well or tube

2 Agglutinated red cell forming a 'carpet' covering the base of the well or tube

APPEARANCE OF THE TEST

Figure XIX.3   TPHA (*Treponema pallidum* haemagglutination) test

Enteric fever

Widal test

1) Make serial dilutions of the patient's serum.
2) Add bacterial suspension:
   H — suspension is a formalinized culture;
   O — suspension is a boiled culture;
   Vi— suspension of formalinized Vi rich bacteria.
3) Incubate H agglutination at 37°C for 2 hours and read after ½ hour on bench.
   Incubate O agglutination at 37°C for 4 hours. Leave overnight at 4°C and read.
   Incubate Vi agglutination at 37°C for 2 hours. Read, after leaving overnight at room temperature.

The interpretation of the results is described in Chapter VII.

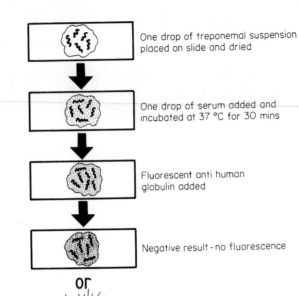

One drop of treponemal suspension placed on slide and dried

One drop of serum added and incubated at 37 °C for 30 mins

Fluorescent anti human globulin added

Negative result - no fluorescence

or

Positive result - fluorescing treponemata

Figure XIX.4   FTA abs (Absorbed Fluorescent Treponemal antibody) test

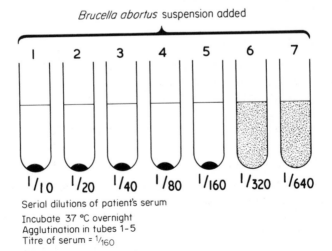

Brucella abortus suspension added

Serial dilutions of patient's serum
Incubate 37 °C overnight
Agglutination in tubes 1-5
Titre of serum = $^1/_{160}$

Figure XIX.5   Direct agglutination test for *Brucella abortus*

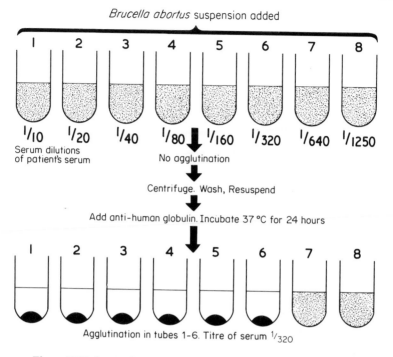

Figure XIX.6   Anti-human globulin (Coombs) test for brucellosis

Brucellosis

1) Direct agglutination test

This detects IgM and is positive in the early disease.
1) Make serial dilutions of patient's serum.
2) Add standard volume *Brucella abortus* suspension.
3) Incubate at 37°C overnight.
4) Examine for agglutination and record titre (Fig. XIX,5).

2) Anti-human globulin (Coombs test)

1) Carry out the test as in the direct agglutination reaction but using a more concentrated suspension.
2) Centrifuge those tubes not showing agglutination and wash the deposit thoroughly.
3) Add anti-human globulin and incubate at 37°C for 24 hours.
4) Read and record titre of agglutination (Fig. XIX,6).

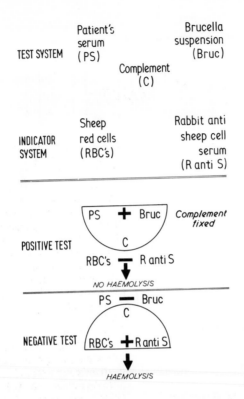

Figure XIX.7   Diagrammatic representation of the use of a complement fixation test in the diagnosis of brucellosis

3) Complement fixation test

1) Add dilutions of patient's serum to brucella suspension with a standard amount of complement.

2) Incubate at 37°C for 1 hour.

3) Sensitize sheep red cells with rabbit anti-sheep cell serum.

4) Add test system to indicator system and incubate at 37°C for 30 minutes.

5) Read and record presence or absence of haemolysisis (Fig. XIX,7).